manhattan medics

the gripping story of the men and women of
Emergency Medical Services who make the
streets of the city their career

manhattan medics

the gripping story of the men and women of
Emergency Medical Services who make the
streets of the city their career

Francis J. Rella, NREMT-P

Elysian Editions
Princeton Book Company, Publishers

Princeton Book Company, Publishers
P.O. Box 831
Hightstown, NJ 08520-0831

Cover design, interior design and composition by Lisa Denham

Library of Congress Cataloging in Publication Data

Rella, Francis J.
    Manhattan medics: the gripping story of the men and women of
    emergency medical services who make the streets of the city their
    career / Francis J. Rella.
    p. cm.
    ISBN 0-87127-258-X   ISBN 0-87127-260-1
    1. Emergency medical technicians—New York (State)—New York.
    2. Emergency medical services—New York (State)—New York.
    3. September 11 Terrorist Attacks, 2001—Personal Narratives.
    4. St. Vincent's Hospital and Medical Center of New York. I. Title.
    RA645.6.N7R45 2003
    362.18'092'297471—dc21
                                                          2003044884

Printed in Canada   6, 5, 4, 3, 2, 1

To my heroes: The firefighters of the FDNY, the police officers of the NYPD and PAPD, the court officers, emergency medical technicians and paramedics who gave their lives on September 11, 2001 and the paramedics of St. Vincent's Hospital, Manhattan.

"We few, we happy few, we band of brothers..."

St. Crispin's Day Speech from Act 4, Scene 3 of Henry V

William Shakespeare

contents

prologue to disaster

About a week before the Towers came down, Carl, Peter, Graciela, and I, all of us City of New York paramedics based at St. Vincent's Hospital, stood at the traffic triangle on Christopher Street and Sixth Avenue for our nightly bitch session.

"I hate the coffee at that place on Fourteenth Street. It tastes like the guy soaks his socks in it," I remarked.

"I know. But I have to visit my people," Carl said.

Carl makes a nightly visit to his local cuties and his entourage. They are scattered at local coffee shops, diners and grocery stores throughout Greenwich Village.

"Can't you visit them without buying their nasty coffee?" I asked.

All of a sudden, Peter turned our attention to the south.

"Look!" he shouted.

As we looked up into the night, we saw the two huge Towers with smoke coming out of them.

"Holy Christ. Do you see what I see?" Carl exclaimed.

"The Towers are on fire!" I gasped. "Let's listen to Citywide."

Citywide is the radio frequency you tune in if the shit really hits the fan. Citywide frequency was silent.

"How about FDNY or PD?" Peter asked.

The fire frequencies were silent. The police frequencies were silent.

"Nothing," Carl said as he switched his attention from one radio to the next, frantically searching for a transmission on any channel.

"Nothing at all? How can that be?" I asked.

"I'm telling you there's nothing," Carl said.

Were we the first ones to see it?

"Guys! It's just a bunch of clouds," said Graciela.

"That's smoke!" Carl fired back.

After a few seconds Peter spoke: "Shit. She's right."

It was the night playing tricks with our eyes. The light from the Twin Towers was reflecting through the clouds, although it looked like a smoldering fire.

I wondered what would have happened if it had been a real fire. Surely the sprinkler systems would kick in. But what a disaster it would be if it really did happen! Could you imagine the amount of casualties? Would our Emergency Medical Services (EMS) system be able to handle it alone? Who would be brave enough or crazy enough to go into the inferno?

Maps

Lower Manhattan

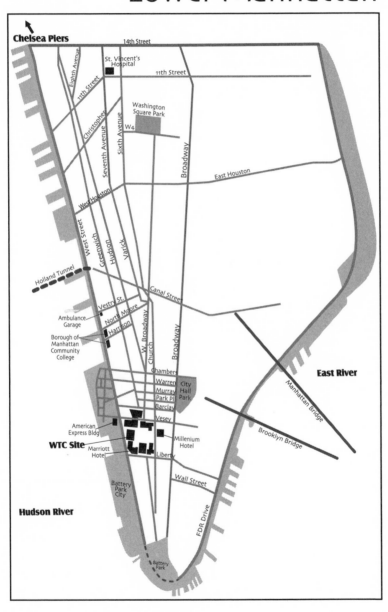

Chelsea Piers
14th Street
St. Vincent's Hospital
11th Street
Eighth Avenue
11th Street
Washington Square Park
Christopher
Seventh Avenue
Sixth Avenue
W4
Broadway
East Houston
West Houston
West Street
Greenwich
Hudson
Varick
Holland Tunnel
Canal Street
Vestry St.
Ambulance Garage
North Moore
Harrison
Borough of Manhattan Community College
W. Broadway
Church
Broadway
Chambers
Warren   City
Murray   Hall
Park Pl   Park
Barclay
Vesey
American Express Bldg
Millenium Hotel
WTC Site Marriott Hotel
Liberty
Battery Park City
Wall Street
FDR Drive
Battery Park

East River
Manhattan Bridge
Brooklyn Bridge

Hudson River

World Trade Center area

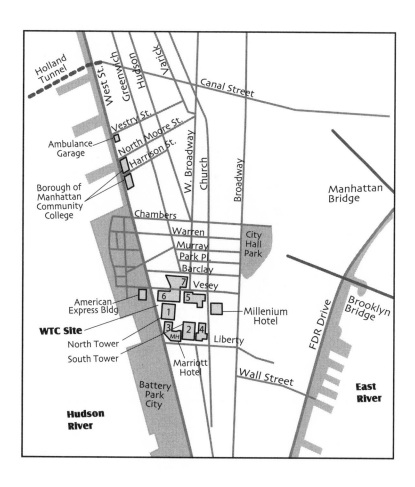

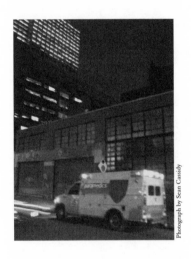

Photograph by Sean Cassidy

1

the days before

For me, the story of the World Trade Center disaster started on Saturday, September 8. That was the last time I got a decent night's sleep.

I work as a paramedic at St. Vincent's Hospital, located in the Greenwich Village/Chelsea section of Lower Manhattan. In New York City, 911 paramedics are either hospital-based or are employed by the Fire Department of New York City (FDNY). Both answer 911 emergency calls. The city does not have enough EMS units, so it subcontracts with the noncity hospitals, such as St. Vincent's, to provide both paramedic and emergency medical technicians.

As a paramedic I am trained to deliver basic first aid to the sick and injured, as well as advanced life support in the form of drug therapy and defibrillation to patients in cardiac arrest. The typical medical calls that we receive are for drug overdose, intoxication, breathing difficulties, and cardiac problems. We also treat traumas: individuals who have been shot, stabbed, or involved in motor vehicle accidents. In most cases paramedics can use medical interventions without consulting with a doctor or hospital. We're the doctors on the street and our ambulance

1

is the hospital.

A few days before the Towers were hit, I was working tour three and the tour one that follows. Tour three is the evening shift, four to midnight. Tour one is midnight to eight—sixteen hours total. It's called a double. With the wrong partner it can feel more like a prison sentence.

On September 8 I was working tour three with Michael Devlin. Michael is a part-time medic and a full-time pain in the ass. Aside from this, Michael is an excellent medic. His one weakness is pretty women. Not that he is unfaithful. He is happily married with three beautiful children and a beautiful wife whom he is crazy about. It's sad, but I do not think his wife knows how much he adores her. But he is faithful to the point of being almost completely sex free.

As I prepared the ambulance for the day's run, Michael gave me his standing orders for the day.

"Clean the bus, then Starbucks, and then off to the girls."

"I thought you are happily married?"

"Like I told you, my wife won't come near me."

"What's up with that?"

"By the time I get the kids to sleep, she's on the phone with her mother. When she gets off the phone, she gets ready for bed."

"And?" I said, waiting for him to continue.

"And what?"

"That's your chance."

"Chance for what?"

"What? Do I have to spell it out for you? You're a young man."

"You don't get it," he said pathetically.

"What do you have to do? Ask permission? It's your wife!"

Michael became silent. I realized that the long and short of it was that he was afraid to approach his spouse about having sex because she might get angry with him. I once heard him talking to his wife on his cell phone, asking her if she would allow him to kiss her when he arrived home from work that night. From his reaction, she obviously said no.

I continued. "Just take her in your arms and kiss her, for Chrissakes." My philosophy is, if somebody is going to be annoyed, it might as well be the other spouse. Why torture yourself? If you are going to get into trouble, there might as well be a reason. I guess Michael has a different opinion.

"What do you think she'll do, sue you?" I asked.

"She would belt me!"

"Come on. Let's go get coffee," I said, shaking my head.

My goal with Michael, other than staying awake through our tour of duty, is to talk as colorfully as I can and attract as many beautiful women to our ambulance as possible. It keeps Michael from being a bitter person and helps me stay awake during the first half of a sixteen-hour shift. All in all, it passes the time with a few laughs.

"This is a long-ass night," I said as we sat in our ambulance, enjoying the view. On that particular night there were lots of beautiful women out and about.

"You want to read some of this?" Michael asked while holding out a portion of *The New York Times*, Sunday Edition.

"I think that there is something sacrilegious about reading the Sunday *Times* on Saturday night. Besides I only read the *Post*." I said, knowing that my comment would annoy him. According to Michael, only subhumans read the *New York Post*. It probably is a rag sheet, but the *Post* has the best sports coverage and theater reviews in New York.

As we sat in our ambulance, a man in his thirties approached our vehicle wearing a Middle-Eastern costume. He had just come out of a bar on Fourteenth Street. I was standing next to the ambulance smoking a cigarette. Cigarette smoke annoyed Michael because it made his uniform smell smoky. His wife would get mad at him because way back when they started dating he promised her that he would not smoke anymore.

"Do you have a cigarette?" the man asked in a thick accent.

"Nice costume," I said as I handed him one from a crumpled pack.

"Thank you," he said, as he lit it. "I do tarot readings. Usually the manager allows me. There is a different man there tonight who doesn't want me hanging around."

"Sorry," I said, as we both blew smoke into the night air.

"Do you want a reading?" he asked.

"No thank you."

"For free!"

"Thanks just the same."

Being a Catholic boy I felt that there was something mysterious and forbidden about the ways of the occult and knew that Michael felt the same.

"Not to insult you but I really don't want to know my future. It would kill my motivation to get out of bed in the morning," I said.

The man finished his cigarette and temporarily became part of our politically incorrect, male chauvinist group, as the three of us watched the beautiful women pass by. Finishing his smoke he said, "Thanks for the cigarette."

I now wonder what would have happened if I had accepted his offer to do my reading. What if he had predicted the Towers' collapse? Could he and I have saved the city?

What would I have done? Would anyone have believed me? I still have a haunting picture in my mind of the tower card from a tarot deck depicting lightning, fire from the sky, people jumping to their death and destruction. In the traditional tarot deck the object that stands under the tower is a structure that closely resembles what was left of the Twin Towers after they were destroyed, a honeycombed piece of metal.

The tarot reader vanished as abruptly as he appeared, and our attention quickly shifted to other things.

As we sat at our assigned corner at Fourteenth Street and Ninth Avenue, dozens of women continued to pass by our ambulance.

"Look at these beauties," I said.

Some of the women stopped for directions and others just to flirt with us. Michael was in his glory. All of a sudden Michael's hormones got the best of him and things began to get out of hand.

"Talk to them, Frank," he said. I hate when people call me Frank. Frank was my father's name. Anyone who is an old friend calls me Frankie, although I know it may seem strange for a man in his forties to be called Frankie.

"You talk to them, Mikey," I said. I know that no one calls him Mikey. Not even his wife. But I think he likes me to call him Mikey because a big grin always comes over his face.

"One of them is smiling at you," he said excitedly.

"She's smiling at you, partner."

"Nobody smiles at me. I am the boy-next-door type. You're the swarthy Latin. They all go crazy for your blue eyes."

I corrected him. "They're green."

"No they aren't," he said, reminding me of my mother who to this day insists that I have blue eyes.

He stuck his face in mine, and after careful examination, which was beginning to make me feel uncomfortable, he said, "They are green. Wow! Are they colored contacts?"

"You're really starting to worry me, partner," I said.

There were a couple of women staring at us, standing a few yards from the ambulance with a larger group. The two women approached the ambulance on my side.

Michael's pupils were about the size of quarters, a typical sympathetic nervous system response, which is usually followed by bronchial dilation, tachycardia, dry mouth, and the inability to urinate or defecate. The typical flight or fight response.

"Can you guys give us a ride?" asked the first woman.

"I'm not going to touch that line with a ten-foot Czechoslo-vakian," I said out loud.

"What?" she asked with a confused look on her face.

"I meant a ten-foot pole," trying to explain my poor excuse for a joke.

"What?" she asked again.

"Skip it," I said.

"See that girl over there?" she continued. There were at least twenty women in the direction she was pointing.

"Oh you mean *that* girl," I said jokingly.

"The blonde in the black dress, silly. We're giving her a bachelorette party. It would be really fun for her to ride in an ambulance with you two handsome men."

"Well, tell her to get really drunk and pass out on the street. Call 911 and we will take you to any hospital in Lower Manhattan," I said.

"You have really nice eyes," she said, completely ignoring my ridiculous response to her ridiculous proposition.

"I told you about your eyes," Michael commented, as if he had uncovered the secret of the ages.

When it comes to my job, I have to adhere strictly to the rules, an attitude that I believed was shared by Michael.

"Come on. It would be fun," she said in a baby voice as she got as close to my face as Michael previously had.

To my amazement, Michael asked, "What are we going to get out of it?"

As my jaw dropped, the second girl asked, "What if we show you our breasts?"

"Just like that?" I asked in complete shock.

Unbelievably, Michael said "OK."

The second girl looked at her friend and asked, "What do you think?"

"He has an honest face," she replied. I didn't know if she was talking about Michael or me. "Wait a minute!" I said.

Before I could sit up, there were four breasts filling the open window on my side of the bus.

This would be a welcome sight to most red-blooded American males—four breasts in your face! However, this was not Mardi Gras in New Orleans. Given the fact that we were in plain view of the general public, in uniform, and sporting a St. Vincent Catholic Medical Centers logo on the side of our vehicle, the only thing I could think of saying was, "Wait a minute!"

7

"Wow!" Michael said quietly.

"Please put those things away," I said, trying to ignore what were now inches away from my face.

Turning to Michael, I saw that he looked as if he had just seen Jesus step off the cross. "Wow!" he repeated.

I said, "Tell them to please put those things away."

"How about our ride?" the first girl asked.

"Hop in the back, ladies!" Michael exclaimed.

"What?" I said.

Michael, being a man of his word and senior partner, ordered me to load the lovely young ladies in the back of the ambulance. "A promise is a promise," he said.

"Have you lost your mind?" I asked.

"My partner will open the back door for you," he announced.

"No. No. This was your idea, partner."

"I'm senior medic, remember? You are the tech."

Looking bewildered, I got out of the vehicle and opened the back door of the ambulance. I tried to appeal to his sense of duty, but he was a man with a vision. After all, he had just seen real breasts! This was probably the biggest thrill he had in months, if not years!

The half dozen or so young ladies of the bridal party turned into nearly twenty people, including various unattached males. Everybody wanted to ride in Michael's ambulance. Michael, still in a daze from seeing live breasts, did not realize that we were about to break an abundant amount of rules, not to mention the basic rules of common decency and good taste.

Just as I was about to triage our "patients" the radio sounded.

"Four King. Ten-thirteen! Ten-thirteen."

A ten-thirteen means an officer or paramedic needed emergency assistance. Usually the crew's getting shot at, stabbed, or getting the hell beat out of them. It is supposed to be used only in an extreme emergency.

I stopped what I was doing and ran to the front of the ambulance as Michael started the engines, sounded the siren and put the emergency lights on. We had a general idea of Four King's location, so we started heading east as we listened to the radio for more details.

We left the bachelorettes behind with a look of bewilderment and anger on their faces.

"Four King, what is your current location?" the dispatcher asked with concern.

"Four King. Four King. Ten-thirteen! Ten-thirteen," the radio sounded.

I typed some information into the onboard computer and it showed that Four King's last location was Second Avenue and East Second Street.

"Two and Two," I said to Michael.

He just nodded his head without any emotion as we hurried to aid the unit in distress. I think Michael might still have been in a daze from the bachelorette breasts, but more probably he was focused on what was happening with Four King. Like all good medics, he was a professional and could turn it back on when he needed to.

"Five William. Show us Sixty-three to Second and Two," Michael said into the microphone.

"Ten-four, Five William."

Every unit in our sector was calling into Central Dispatch and saying that they were on the way to help Four King.

"All units. Stand by until we can ascertain the problem," ordered the dispatcher.

Michael ignored the order and continued to proceed to Second Avenue and East Second street.

As we drew closer to the scene, the voice of one of the emergency medical technicians (EMTs) from Four King was heard on the radio.

"Cancel the units, Central. We're alright."

Michael gave me a look of astonishment. There was a long silence over the radio, and then Michael keyed the microphone.

"Central, this is Five William. What is the status of Four King?"

"Stand by, Five William," the dispatcher replied.

After another long silence, the radio sounded. "No further assistance is needed. Conditions Zero Four is on the scene. There is no danger to the unit."

"What the hell is that about?" I said out loud.

"I don't know. But I'm going to find out," said Michael as he stopped the ambulance and fished his cell phone from his breast pocket. Frantically he dialed some numbers and called Central Dispatch. After speaking to the tour commander he closed the cover and shoved the tiny phone back into his pocket.

"Someone was getting belligerent with them," he said in amazement.

"So they call a thirteen?" I asked.

"They got a conditions boss with them right now, probably chewing them another orifice."

"Let's just go and kick their ass," I said.

"I'm glad that they're alright, but it was a damn stupid thing to do."

I shook my head and added, "Almost as stupid as if we had taken all those girls for a ride!"

"Almost," said Michael with a smirk on his face.

Later that night, as we drove to the garage for the change of shift, Michael had an anxious look on his face.

"You're not going to tell anyone about the breasts, are you?" he asked nervously, as if he had just been caught looking at a girlie magazine.

I said, "Michael. I never kiss and tell."

Relief came to his worried face.

"I kiss and exaggerate."

2
9/09

I'm beat," I announced.

"No problem. We'll get our coffee and go nest," Peter replied.

Peter and I began the midnight-to-eight shift with every intention of getting some rest. The good thing about the night shift is that you can get some rest if it's not too busy. The bad thing is that every time you really want to rest, it gets really busy.

On that particular night we started heading towards the hospital by way of a coffee shop. It was our normal routine. We would check out the ambulance, get a cup of coffee, and go to the hospital to see who the attending physician was for the night.

A call came over the radio for a patient in respiratory arrest.

"Five William," the dispatcher's voice announced.

"Five Willie," Peter replied.

"Proceed to Two Four and Nine. Back up Five Adam for the unconscious. Possible overdose in respiratory arrest," said the dispatcher.

"Five Willie. Sixty-three," Peter said as he pushed the various switches that lit the emergency lights.

Five Adam, the EMT Basic Life Support Unit (BLS), had called Central Dispatch for paramedic assistance, and we arrived on the scene within two minutes. It was outside a club, and a young man lay on the stretcher and backboard, holding his breath and clamping his eyes shut.

Peter and I peeked in the back of the ambulance and started to inquire about his condition from the two FDNY EMTs who were already on the scene. His condition appeared to be "feigning lark," which means faking fainting.

Peter asked, "What's the deal with this guy?"

"He got punched by the bouncer in the club, walked up to our bus, and passed out. Now he's not breathing," replied Ace.

Richie "Ace" Acevedo was an old-time EMT with a dozen years of experience on the street. He worked the overnight shift on Five Adam, which was our usual BLS backup unit.

Peter got onboard and started to evaluate the patient and all of us agreed that he was pretty much full of crap, pretending to be passed out. I followed Peter onto the bus, as several police officers were looking on from the street.

"He's belly breathing," Peter said.

"What the hell is that?" Ace asked.

"He's holding his breath every time we check him out, but his belly keeps moving up and down," I explained.

As Peter started to do a head to toe evaluation, a call came over the radio that an Advanced Life Support (ALS) unit was needed in our area for a pediatric anaphylactic shock, which meant a child was having a severe life-threatening allergic reaction.

"C'mon buddy. I have no time for this. Stop playing games with us!" Peter said loudly.

I proceeded to administer the hand test. If a patient is truly unconscious, when you lift his arm straight up in the air and let it fall, his hand will strike his face. If he is faking it, the patient will let the hand and arm fall to his chest or midsection. I administered the hand test several times and each time the patient avoided hitting himself in the face. This was a bullshit 911 call.

While we were playing games with our patient, we were possibly needed by a child that might have been unable to breathe.

A bystander once asked me, "Aren't all emergency calls important?"

"Yes," I replied. "However, not all 911 calls are emergency calls." But once we are on a call, regulations say that we have to stay on a call.

As our frustration mounted, I announced to the patient that I was going to stick a big needle in his arm and it was going to hurt a lot. That usually wakes them up if they are faking it. As I started to prepare his arm for the IV he began to be combative with Peter. Peter is a good-natured guy, but he has very little patience for this sort of thing. This guy was clearly playing a game with us.

"I'm gonna have to give you drugs that you probably don't need," I added.

The patient continued to keep his eyes tightly shut. When he could no longer hold his breath, he finally exhaled and started breathing quickly.

"You want the big needle?" Peter asked in a loud voice.

"Give me the big needle," I replied loudly enough for the patient and the cops standing outside the vehicle to hear.

The patient still did not open his eyes as Peter handed me a normal-size syringe.

"OK, sir. Here it comes," Peter said as the cops chuckled at our theatrics.

The patient opened one eye long enough to see the syringe coming at him and started to flail about, trying to hit both of us.

"OK, knock it off before we get PD to put you in cuffs," Peter shouted.

While Peter and the crew from Five Adam along with two police officers tried to restrain him, I put down the syringe and looked at the patient's eyes with a penlight.

"I think we should give him some Narcan just in case."

"Really?" Peter asked with a surprised look on his face.

"His pupils look a little constricted. I don't know if it's the light in the bus or if he might be on something. Hard to tell. In any case it couldn't hurt."

Naloxone (Narcan) is an inert drug. It is completely harmless and it only works as an antidote if a patient has taken opiates.

"OK. We'll hold him down," Peter said to me.

"Look, sir. If you don't level with us you're going to get the needle," I said again in a loud voice.

I drew up two milligrams of Narcan and gave it intramuscularly. The sting from the needle made the patient open his eyes and it became clear that he didn't have constricted pupils, so he was probably not on opiates. As he shouted at us, the smell of alcohol wafted from his mouth.

I got an IV in his arm in case we had to give him other medications. I tested his blood sugar level and it was normal. Also, nothing indicated that he had altered consciousness due to a head injury. As we rolled to the hospital he was still thrashing about, obviously pissed that we were giving him medications.

No sooner did we clean our ambulance than a car pulled up alongside.

"Excuse me. A girl got hit by a car," said the driver.

"Where?" I asked.

"Fourteenth and Seventh," he replied.

We called the dispatcher over the radio and put ourselves on the job.

"Central. This is Zero Five William. Put us on the job for a pedestrian struck on Fourteen and Seven."

"Ten-four, Five William." Ten-four is radio code for "Yes I understand."

Without the protection of a police vehicle to divert traffic, Peter and I ran into the middle of Seventh Avenue and stabilized the young female patient. Cars were not stopping and came very close to running us over despite our flashing lights.

"Goddamn cars!" Peter said.

"Pete, get the stretcher and long board and be careful, for Chrissakes," I said.

We put the patient in our ambulance and started two large bore IV lines in her arms.

"How was the bachelorette party?" I asked.

"It was fun," she replied.

"What is she talking about?" Peter asked.

"I'll tell you later," I said.

The young woman was the guest of honor at the bachelorette party. Her beautiful blonde hair was now stained with blood and her eyes were blackened from tear-soaked mascara. One of the girls who displayed her breasts to Michael and me was now sitting in the back of our ambulance holding her friend's hand.

"What happened?" I asked.

"I was crossing the street and this guy ran the red light," said the patient.

"He hit her and kept right on going," her friend added.

"Son of a bitch," Peter said as he exited the back of the ambulance.

"Don't worry, we'll take care of you," I said.

"I'm getting married tomorrow," she said.

I smiled at her and avoided her eyes as I continued to work. I called to Peter who was now in the front of the ambulance. "Let's roll, partner."

3
9/10–9/11

I was off from work on Sunday night and returned on Monday evening for another double shift—the tour three shift on the tenth of September and Tuesday morning tour one on the eleventh of September.

I arrived at the ambulance garage at four o'clock on Monday afternoon on West Street, a few blocks north of the World Trade Center in Lower Manhattan.

I really had not gotten any sleep. I was wound up and a little jumpy. I was trying to strike a balance between my personal life and my work life, and I was having lots of problems with both.

In 1996, after the birth and death of our only son, my marriage started falling apart. The relationship I had with Tammy, my wife of thirteen years, always had been distant. We were from very different backgrounds. She was from a midwestern Protestant family and I was an Italian-American Catholic from New York. I always made the error of mistaking her unperturbed behavior for stoicism. Our inability at times to discern each other's strengths and weaknesses, in addition to a heart attack I had in 1998, caused us to grow further apart. Our estrangement turned into a legal separation and eventually we filed for divorce.

Despite our separation, I still lived in the same house, saw my daughters every day, and was a full-time father. My regular tour of duty was the midnight-to-eight shift. At times I worked double shifts, which began at four in the afternoon. I would usually work a double only on weekends. If I worked a double during the week, I would not leave for work until my children arrived home safely.

Tammy was home for them before school and I was with them after school. We were both there at dinner time. That was the only good thing about working nights: I was available for my children every day when they stepped off the school bus. I could also be with them until they went to sleep. In fact, the only time I was not there was when they were sleeping. The trade-off was that I had a limited amount of time to sleep. At the same time I was trying to get work in show business. This was one more thing to stress about.

It was Monday night and all the secret squirrels and EDPs (emotionally disturbed persons) were still recovering from the weekend. Weeknights were usually very quiet, and I really needed some quiet time. I had a lot of things to take care of on Tuesday and I needed a day off. I wanted to pay a visit to my chiropractor for an acute back problem and I had to sit for two nursing exams.

As I entered the garage to change ambulances and pick up Peter, Jim Amato, the ambulance supervisor, was getting ready to go home. Jim was small in stature but he had the heart of a giant. He was a tough Italian who resembled Napoleon. Jim could not be bullshitted, although he was king of the bullshit artists. His methods of covering open ambulance shifts were like those of a used car salesman. If you needed a day off, somehow Jim would convince you to work three days in return and you would wind up thanking him.

Jim was always willing to work out problems in the schedule and kept mandations to a minimum. A mandation is being required to work an extra eight hours when your relief calls in sick. Getting mandated was especially disturbing when you barely got any sleep prior to your shift. It usually meant you were up for more than twenty-four hours before you finally got off from work. It was not really a good idea either in terms of patient care or in terms of your health. Sixteen hours was long enough to spend on an ambulance, sometimes dealing with life and death decisions.

"Jim. I need a favor," I said.

"Don't tell me. You need a day off," he said, not looking up from his stack of papers.

"I need to take an emergency personal day tomorrow night. Urgent personal business."

"Tomorrow? That's really short notice," he said. I did not answer. "Do me a favor. Leave a message on Bill Batista's voice mail. He's the supervisor tomorrow. Let him handle it. I'm off for four days," he continued. He handed me a stack of papers. "Here. Sign these and date them," he ordered.

"Nine-eleven," I said as I wrote 9/11 on each page. "How weird is that?"

"Pretty weird," he answered.

Peter and I headed towards the hospital to begin our tour of duty. We drove around the neighborhood but all the regulars were nowhere to be found. The only one that we saw was Ronald Reagan and he was surprisingly sober.

Ronald Reagan is an indigent who is a chronic alcoholic somewhere in his fifties. One time he was so intoxicated that his heart stopped.

A St. Vincent's paramedic crew brought him back to life. He spent two months in the Medical Intensive Care Unit at a cost of thousands of taxpayer dollars. On the day he left the hospital he was clean-shaven, had new clothes and was amazingly coherent. He had a new outlook on life, having been brought back from the dead, and twenty dollars in his pocket. Ronald Reagan was indeed a new man.

Four hours later the same crew that brought him back from full cardiac arrest two months before picked him up on the street, covered in feces and as drunk as a skunk.

My first encounter with him was when I was a brand-new medic. He was reluctant to go to the hospital.

"I'm not going to the hospital and you can't make me," he stated.

"Listen, Mr. President, it's time for your annual checkup at Bethesda Naval Hospital."

"But I don't want to go on the ambulance."

"That's not an ambulance."

"It's not?"

"Certainly not, Mr. President. That's Air Force One. And that young gentleman standing there is a Secret Service agent." Without hesitation he marched onto the ambulance. I questioned him further once we were both onboard. "Is there someone we can contact once we get to the hospital?"

"You can call my bitch of a wife," he growled.

"Don't tell me. Her name is Nancy!"

"How did you know?"

"Lucky guess."

Since then I only refer to him as "Mr. President."

In the early morning hours of 9/11, Peter and I saw him sitting on a bench outside the Fourteenth Street subway station as sober as a minister. As we passed by, I yelled out of the window, "Mr. President, how are you doing tonight?" He just smiled and waved.

"Do you want to go to the hospital?" Peter asked. Ronald Reagan was looking particularly stinky.

"No. No," he called back in a commanding voice, as the elder statesman that he was. "But thanks for your support."

"Damn," Peter remarked. "I feel like giving him five bucks and telling him to go buy a bottle."

We drove around for a good long while, and just as we were going to find a quiet spot to rest the radio blared.

"Five William," said Central Dispatch.

"Five Willie. Go," said Peter.

"Five William. Proceed to Two-three and Seven. Ninety-year-old female, difficulty in breathing."

When we got to the location, a high-rise apartment, we found a very lucid lady with her son.

"How long have you had problems with your breathing?" I asked, as Peter put a blood pressure cuff on her arm.

"For about ten years," she answered.

"No. I mean tonight, ma'am?"

"I don't have any problems tonight."

"Didn't you tell me that you were feeling sick?" the son said, trying to coach his mother.

"OK, we are going to examine you and take you to the hospital because they might have to do some tests," I explained.

"I want her to go to Columbia Presbyterian. All her doctors are there," the son ordered.

"That's a little far," Peter said.

After doing a quick physical exam on the mother, I turned my attention back to the son. "Considering your mother's age, she should probably go to the nearest 911 hospital. Broadway and One-sixty-eight Street is way out of our area."

"No, no, no, no, no!" the son said excitedly. "Columbia Presbyterian on Two hundred and Twentieth Street!"

"Allen Pavilion?" I asked.

"No way! That's two hundred blocks away!" Peter said.

"When I called 911 I was told that you would take my mother to any hospital I asked. Don't you ambulance drivers have to go where I say? It's not like you are doing anything important this morning!"

"Look, I'm leaving for the Hamptons for four days, and if she needs to be hospitalized and I am not here, she could die. As long as she's feeling sick, it's better that she is with her own doctors."

"So, basically this whole thing is bullshit. There's nothing wrong with your mom. You want the system to baby-sit her while you're away," I said.

"You have to take her. You know the system."

"I'm not going to stand here and argue with you all night. Tell you what, if the medical control doctor says we can go up there then we'll take the drive. If not, you go where we say, otherwise we call PD," I said.

Peter and I were both sure that considering the patient's age we would be directed to the nearest 911 hospital by telemetry.

Much to our surprise, the physician at FDNY said, "Sure, go ahead." So off we went two hundred blocks uptown.

4
daybreak, 9/11

Nothing beats a long transport in the back of an ambulance. It reminded me of my first days as a paramedic. When I suffered through working as a transport paramedic I lived on Bayer aspirin and Rolaids.

I was ready to vomit when we finally got to Columbia Presbyterian, Allen Pavilion, and Peter had no idea where the hell he was. The patient's son directed Peter into the hospital entrance and we brought our patient to the nurse's station on the stretcher. The pretty middle-aged African-American triage nurse looked as confused as we did when we told her we were from St. Vincent's Hospital.

"What are you boys doing up here? Are you lost? Is this a transfer? Nobody called us," she said in rapid succession.

"No. This is a 911 call."

"And you brought her here?" she said as she sucked her cheek and made a disapproving sound.

"Family member request," Peter added.

"And telemetry approved it?" she asked.

"Yes ma'am."

"Is there a problem? Her doctor knows that she is coming here," the son said.

The veteran nurse knew that something was not quite right.

"You know, you shouldn't be abusin' the system, sir. These two good looking white boys don't need to be travelin' up here. They got their own work to do downtown.

"Don't worry, sir," she continued. "We'll take good care of your momma. You can have a seat and enjoy some of the local color."

She made the son go to the waiting room while we transferred our patient to a hospital bed. In the waiting room was a collection of skells, drunks, and crackheads. The son looked like he felt out of place wearing a polo shirt, khaki pants, and penny loafers. Suddenly his arrogance was replaced by fear.

I dropped off the paperwork at the admit desk, and as I helped Peter push the stretcher to the ambulance we saw the son being harassed by a Sterno bum.

Several minutes after we left the hospital, Peter looked at me and admitted, "I hate to say it, but I think I'm lost."

"No problem. Just head south towards the Towers," I replied.

It was a beautiful quiet morning, and as we pulled up to St. Vincent's it was just getting light. We saw the flag outside of the hospital blowing in the soft summer breeze. It reminded me of the first lines of the "Star Spangled Banner."

Peter and I sat in front of the hospital for a while, and there was a strange quiet that we both remarked about that still haunts me.

"Hey, Pete, do you notice anything strange?" I asked.

Peter thought for a moment. It was uncanny, but we could almost always read each other's thoughts. We would often finish each other's sentences.

"Yeah, no cabs," he said.

Usually, Seventh Avenue is packed with tons of cabs anytime, day or night. I once counted fifty cabs in one minute and that was at four in the morning. That day, September 11, 2001, at seven a.m., there were none.

Our shift was almost over and we decided that it would be foolish to get any rest.

"I'm tired. Let's get some liquid crack," said Peter.

We headed over to Casa d'Oro to get some Spanish black coffee. It could wake up a corpse.

"I'm buying," I offered.

"You bought last time."

"No, you did."

"No way. You did. My turn!"

Peter and I would always argue about who bought last. Whoever got to the cashier first would pay for meals and coffee. I guess it was because we both grew up poor, with mothers who were the sole support of our families. Now that we had a little money, we were going to be the "big spenders" that we could never be as kids.

As we passed Fourteenth Street and Eighth Avenue, I exclaimed, "Look at this shit!"

"What the hell are we rolling up on?" Peter asked.

"Zero Five William, show us flagged at Fourteen and Eight for the intox," I said into the walkie-talkie.

"Ronald freaking Reagan!" Peter said as we exited the vehicle.

"C'mon, Mr. President. Time to go the White House. We don't want to worry Nancy," I said as I turned him over gently. He was lying face down, passed out on the sidewalk.

We were less than thrilled. This is a lousy last job but at least we would not get banged with a late job. Peter and I are the kings of late jobs. I think Peter's wife believes that we always get late jobs so we can hang out together for an extra hour. A few days before, we were sent to the Twin Towers and did not get off from work until after nine a.m.

I always hated going to a job in the Towers. The elevators would take you up fifty floors at a time. It was always an uncomfortable ride. The only pleasant thing was the Port Authority police officers who accompanied us. There was one guy in particular who would always tell us how much he loved St. Vincent's paramedics. "I love you guys: you're the best!"

I later saw his photograph hanging up at the police memorial at Liberty Street, one of the missing.

By the time we got Ronald Reagan onto the ambulance, drove to the hospital, did the paperwork and cleaned up it was already close to eight o'clock. We then drove to our ambulance garage, which sat about eight city blocks from the World Trade Center.

It was a little after eight a.m. when Peter shut the engine off. The change of crew was already getting their ambulance together. Ned Edwards, a long-time veteran of EMS, and Andrew Johns, a medic for six years, were like clockwork as far as relieving the previous crew was concerned. Also, if they were your shift change there was very little chance of getting mandated because they hardly ever called in sick. They were Five William tour two, which runs from eight a.m. until four p.m.

We all made small talk as they readied their ambulance and we put ours away.

"Oh, shit! We have to go to choir practice!" I suddenly said.

"No. I forgot to tell you. It's called off," Peter said.

Choir practice was the term we used for meeting together and getting drunk. It is pretty nasty to drink in the early morning hours, but it's really the nighttime for tour one people.

"I can't say I'm disappointed. I've already been up for twenty hours. I have the worst migraine of my life," I said.

"You want some aspirin?" Peter asked.

"I want some sleep."

"I feel your pain, brother."

"You want to go for breakfast?"

"I would, but I gotta get home to the missus. She has a honey-do list waiting for me," Peter said, annoyed.

"A farmer's work is never done," Ned said without looking up from his work.

Peter had just bought a farm in upstate New York.

"I'll see you Wednesday night. I'm taking tonight off," I said.

5
rush hour

When the first plane hit, I was on the road somewhere in Central New Jersey. Usually I listen to an all-news radio station on my way home from work, but with my migraine I just wanted to drive in silence with my own thoughts. My mind was preoccupied with how crappy my life was: my marriage problems and the feeling that I had a failed life. I was really feeling sorry for myself and I could not shake the mood of depression that was probably brought on by being without sleep for so long and not eating in sixteen hours, as well as being in physical pain.

I was on the verge of quitting my job as a paramedic. I never wanted to be a full-time paramedic, just as I never wanted to be a full-time teacher.

I spent the early part of my adult life as a professional actor. After getting married, I spent the next thirteen years teaching high school students in what was supposed to be a temporary job. Circumstances and lack of free time prevented me from pursuing a career as an actor again, although I occasionally worked professionally. My plan was to work as a medic part-time and spend the rest of my time looking for acting jobs. I wanted desperately to go back into show business and I believed that being a medic would make it possible, since the hours did not interfere with auditions. On paper, being a paramedic looked like it would be a great day job. The reality was that extensive debt forced me into voluntary servitude having to work countless overtime shifts on top of being mandated. The fatigue alone was beginning to wear me down, although fatigue was no stranger to me.

At the end of my service in the Gulf War, I had come down with mysterious medical symptoms. After going to countless doctors, initially I was diagnosed as having Epstein-Barr Virus/Chronic Fatigue Syndrome. Given my medical and military history, what was finally decided was that I was suffering from Gulf War Syndrome.

Then at the age of thirty-eight I suffered a massive heart attack, which was due to a combination of bad genes, an unhealthy lifestyle, and too much stress. Although I had a medical background as a navy hospital corpsman, having a heart attack was the reason why I finally became interested in a career as a paramedic.

As far as stress was concerned, paramedicine offered no relief. In a way it was less stressful than running a high school fine arts program, but I was beginning to feel the effects of the everyday unconscious strain.

So as I drove home to Old Bridge, New Jersey, there was nothing to tip me off that anything was wrong. Traffic heading into New York was normally congested, but nothing looked like it was out of the ordinary. On the last few minutes of the trip my cell phone started to ring nonstop.

Caller ID told me that the calls were from my friend Tara Cornetto. Tara is an actress in New York City. I had not spoken to her for a while and I was going to call her as soon as I got home. I just let my voicemail pick up her calls because the pain in my head was making me nauseous. I had to use all my energy to concentrate on driving and staying awake. As I pulled into the driveway of my house, I received a call from the ambulance office. I supposed it was Bill Batista telling me that I could not have the personal day that I requested. I really did not want to deal with it at the moment. I was so tired that all I wanted to do was sleep.

Once I stopped the car, I called my voicemail and Tara's voice sounded panicked. I could not really understand what she was talking about. Something about "staying out of the city." Something else about a "terrorist attack." What the hell was she so upset about? It really did not make any sense. The last message cleared it up.

My supervisor, Bill, left me the following voicemail: "A plane crashed into the World Trade Center. I'm not bullshitting; it's really bad. I need all the medics to come in. It's a total recall situation. Call the office."

Total recall? A plane crashing into the Trades at this hour? There have to be hundreds of casualties, I thought.

I quickly went into the house to see if my daughters, Rose and Maria, were there. It was around 8:40 and I hoped they did not go to school.

"Where are the girls?" I said as I walked in the door. Tammy was on the phone and the television was turned on. She quickly hung up the phone and was crying. "They're in school," she replied.

"What the hell is going on?" I said.

"A plane crashed into the World Trade Center," she said as tears ran down her cheeks. I have known Tammy since she was nineteen years old. Generally she is a very unflappable person, which is the thing I admire most about her. It has enabled her to face true sadness and adversity and carry on. Even with the death of our only son she shed no tears publicly. I knew if she was crying that something was really, really wrong.

I stood there for a few seconds in disbelief as we both watched the TV. One of the Towers had smoke coming out of it. I called the office and told them I was on my way.

"I gotta go right back," I said as I walked toward the door.

6
total recall

I jumped into my car and rushed back toward the city, tuned into the news. The newscasters didn't seem to know anything other than that a plane had crashed into one of the Towers. I drove at lightning speed in anticipation of the worst. The turnpike was backed up for miles. I had no emergency lights or sirens, but I got into the service lane and flashed my high beams, beeped my horn, and held my badge out of the window to move cars out of my way, but with little success.

Out of the blue, an unmarked car passed my vehicle with its emergency lights flashing and a siren blaring. I pulled in back of it and followed its lead. Drivers were not eager to let cars get ahead of them during rush hour, but I managed to get as far as the Lincoln Tunnel exit of the turnpike without any delay. The Holland Tunnel exit was completely inaccessible. I never knew who the man was that was blazing the trail for me, but I waved to him in thanks as he exited. I will never forget his face or his resolve.

While I was making my way to the tunnel, I realized that my gas gauge was past empty. The last thing I wanted to have happen was to run out of gas on the day of the worst MCI on record. An MCI is a mass casualty incident where five or more people are injured.

I pulled off the highway and drove into a gas station on the service road. I coaxed the attendant to serve me first. Since I was in uniform and flashing my badge he complied immediately.

From that vantage point, I could see the Towers. The North Tower had smoke pouring out of the upper floors. It was around nine a.m. I still didn't realize what was going on and the news radio was no help. At that point all that I thought happened was that a plane had accidentally crashed into the building. A plane. Not a jet filled with passengers and a full tank of fuel.

When I got back on the highway, emergency vehicles were heading toward the tunnel. There were drivers in uniform and cars with uniforms hanging in the back seats. We were all trying to get around the civilian cars, which, as usual, jammed the access to the tunnel. Men in civilian clothes, standing on the road with badges hanging from their shirts, were diverting cars, trying to make a path in one of the lanes so emergency workers could pass.

My sense of urgency was relieved when a Port Authority police officer waved me through as I was coming down the home stretch about a mile away from the tunnel.

It was eerie, being the lone car in the normally crowded tunnel. What the hell was going on?

I exited and drove toward the West Side Highway, going through red lights and hoping to find a cop car to get me to my ambulance garage. I was on Twenty-third Street and West Street, passing the Chelsea Piers, with a little less than a mile to go in order to reach my garage on Vestry and West Streets, and there were no police vehicles in sight. The streets were virtually abandoned. The only pedestrians were civilians walking in the opposite direction, away from West Street, and a couple of joggers completely oblivious to what was going on. Joggers for Chrissakes! Only in New York!

I blasted my horn as if sounding a charge toward a battlefield.

7
race to the towers

Farther down West Street, dozens of cars were speeding toward the Towers, and men in uniform waved us on. I had one hand on the wheel and the other holding my badge out of the window. As I approached the ambulance garage, I saw a sea of people walking calmly in our direction. They looked like they had been through a war. There had to be thousands of them, ten or more abreast, walking from the Trade Center all the way up to the ambulance garage. There was fear in their faces, but no one looked panicked. They looked like they were all helping and comforting each other as they walked. It was around 9:30 a.m.

West Street was full of emergency vehicles in a long line, stacked up and all facing south, waiting to converge upon the Towers. I made it as far as the garage on the opposite side of the street, but I could not turn my car around. I pulled in back of another vehicle parked on the street by the center divider. God knows if it was going to get towed away, but that did not seem important. All I wanted to do was get an ambulance and head down to the Towers.

As I got out of my car, I could see that smoke was now coming out of both Towers. Holy shit, I thought, this is really going to be bad!

I jumped over the divider and walked through the open doors

of the ambulance garage past Desmond Engle and Joe Moffitt, two veteran medics who were parking their cars.

"What the hell is going on? How did the South Tower catch fire?" I asked.

"Another plane hit it. Move your car off the road!" Desmond ordered. I just kept walking past him.

Sometime during the trip back into the city, I heard on the radio that a plane had crashed into the Pentagon and it all clicked in my head. This was a damn deliberate act! America was being attacked on her own soil!

I hurried to the drug cabinet and got a set of narcotics out of the lockbox and grabbed a radio. There were a few medics scurrying about looking for supplies and loading up their self-chosen ambulances.

"We gotta get every dust mask we can," said Chester.

"Take as many O_2 tanks as the bus can hold!" shouted Esteban.

"Guys, guys. Leave some supplies for the rest of us! You're not the only medic unit going to the Towers," Joe barked.

They just kept taking things, not listening to or acknowledging anyone. It was as if they were shell shocked.

They only briefly snapped back into reality when they realized that I had a lit cigarette dangling from my mouth.

"Put that out!" they both shouted.

"What the hell for?" I asked as I looked for an available ambulance.

"We got the onboard O_2 tank running," Esteban said.

"What the hell for?" I asked again.

"In case it's a chemical attack!" Esteban answered.

"And we've been taking oral antibiotics, too!" Chester added.

"What, have you guys lost your friggin' marbles!" I said. "If your rig catches fire, you'll be blown to kingdom come!"

Had the whole world gone mad? Chemical and biological attacks. This was Manhattan for Godsakes!

They went back into their own world and continued to scurry around the ambulance garage.

Desmond Engle said to me, "You stay here. Joe and I are paired up together."

"As soon as I get a partner, I'm out of here. I'm taking seventeen-fifty-one," I announced.

"Kendra. You're with me," I said. Kendra Camp nodded in agreement. Kendra was tall with striking good looks.

Initially, and in a strange way, I was comforted by the idea that if I was going to die it might as well be with a beautiful woman.

As I waited for the other ambulances to move out of the way, I called the paramedic office at the hospital and asked them if the garage could be used as a triage center for any walking wounded. Medic supervisor Gabe Abrams gave me the green light. Arriving after me was one of the new medics, Marco Farina, who was without a partner, so I passed the word to him.

"Until you get a partner and relief, you're in charge of the triage center on orders of the supervisor." I made it clear that he was not, under any circumstances, allowed to leave the garage until he was properly relieved.

As I pulled the ambulance out and joined the line, I saw a former classmate of mine, Joe Lauria, who was working EMS for FDNY up in the South Bronx when the Towers were hit. At the end of his tour of duty, his unit was sent to Lower Manhattan. His rig was parked in front of our ambulance garage. We hugged each other.

"Thank God you are all right," he said.

One of the main thoughts in my mind was of my partner Peter and his whereabouts. He had to have heard about this, I thought. What if he got here before me? What if he's at the Towers already? I started becoming really impatient. I was sitting in a line waiting to go into combat and my best friend could be in harm's way. I knew Peter would be in the thick of it if he were there. I didn't really mind getting killed; that's part of the job. But I would not want Peter to die alone. Shit. Why are we just sitting here?

What of the other crews? What about Andrew Johns and Ned? They were our relief.

It was then that I saw the crew from Seven King. Diego was standing by his ambulance, facing north on West Street. He was smoking a cigarette and had the thousand-mile stare.

"Were you down there?" I asked.

"It's bad, pop. Really bad."

"Thank God you're OK."

Bobbie came up from behind me. Bobbie Pederson was Diego's partner on Seven King. Seven King was one of the St. Vincent's ambulance units that was on duty when the Towers first got hit. "Where are you going?" she asked with concern. I just looked at her.

"Please don't go down there. You can't go down there. There are people dying down there," she said as she pounded my chest with her fists.

"Bobbie. Bobbie. That is what we do," I said. A moment of silence was replaced by a high-pitched sound, followed by the sound of a freight train and, finally, what felt like an earthquake.

"What the hell happened?" I asked out loud as Bobbie continued to hold onto me. We looked south and saw that there was a hole in the sky and a big empty space where one of the Towers once stood. "Holy Christ! How could that be?" After all, planes have hit buildings before! "Where did the building go? Why didn't it topple? Was the plane carrying a payload? Did someone bomb us?"

One of the male medics fell to his knees and started to weep openly. "All the guys from Beekman Hospital were down there. They're all dead," he said, covering his face with his hands.

All of us wanted to get down to the remaining Tower in a hurry. People cried and held onto each other. Soot and dust covered the morning sky. We were close enough to see what happened, but too far away to make out things clearly. All we knew was that our friends and brothers were down there and a building fell on top of them.

The ambulance crews hurried back to their vehicles and started to jockey them into position, ready to swoop down upon the Towers.

"Everyone stand by. Do not proceed to the Towers. Stand by," an FDNY-EMS officer shouted over a bullhorn, sensing that chaos was about to ensue.

Just then, an overwhelming smell of gas filled the air. "A gas leak! Holy shit!" We were going to get blown to perdition before we had the chance to help save some lives. This would be a shitty way to go! Kendra and I jumped into our vehicle and headed north in full retreat. Suddenly, I was a general leading the charge, but it was in the wrong damn direction!

I waved my arm frantically at the other crews and gave them the military sign of a gas attack, hoping they would understand me. I then grabbed the onboard microphone and broadcasted: "Gas, gas. Evacuate the area," over and over. I saw the other crews getting in their vehicles and following behind us.

The dispatcher on the radio told all units to proceed to the Chelsea Piers up on Twenty-third Street.

"All units proceed to Chelsea Piers. New triage area is going to be located at the Chelsea Piers," the dispatcher repeated.

Those in command were setting up a staging area and a triage center. There were going to be thousands of casualties for sure!

As Kendra and I headed toward the piers, the divider between the highway was crowded with civilians all cheering and waving us on. Someone held a sign up that said, "Heroes Highway." For that one moment in time, New York was a small town and we were its only hope of getting through this bloodbath. We were the knights of New York.

Kendra started to get very anxious. She lived in the Chelsea neighborhood, and her kids were without their mother.

"I have to get to my kids," she said.

"Take it easy."

"I just want to get them into a car and get them out of the city."

"The city is shut down. No vehicles in or out. I barely made it back."

"Just get me to my apartment."

"Listen Kendra, I promise we'll go there. First let's get to the hospital and tell them that we are on the street. As soon as we do that I'll drive you to your apartment." I wanted to find out about Peter and the rest of our crews. I wanted to drive Kendra home and make sure that she got there safely. I was not going to be in the rear waiting for patients at the damn Chelsea Piers or sitting on West Street waiting to get blown up! I needed to get to the front lines.

By the time we pulled up to St. Vincent's, a minute or two later, Kendra was inconsolable. She really is an excellent medic, but she was a mother, first, and I do not know how I would have behaved in a similar circumstance. My daughters were safe in New Jersey, after all.

As we drove down Seventh Avenue, St. Vincent's was already deployed. Hospital beds lined the sidewalk and there were dozens of people in position waiting desperately for the first ambulance to arrive. Little did I know that we were the first ambulance that reached St. Vincent's after the hospital set up for mass casualties.

"What did you bring us?" asked Nick Terranova, paramedic supervisor.

"Nothing. I just wanted to stop here and tell you we are heading down there," I replied.

Kendra jumped out of the vehicle, wearing the emergency helmet and carrying the second helmet in her hand, not realizing what she was doing.

"I gotta go."

"Wait a minute, Kendra."

"Sorry. I have to get to my kids."

I understood her motive completely. At that moment, however, I was without a partner and without a helmet.

8

charging south

Go ahead. Do what you have to do today. There will be no way to talk to you by radio," said Bill Batista, ambulance department manager.

Basically, my supervisors gave me the green light to act on my own authority.

"You got another partner for me, and a couple of helmets?" I asked them.

Seeing Nick Terranova standing close to the open door with an anxious look on his face, I shouted, "Hop on!"

As soon as Nick boarded he shouted back, "Let's go!"

"Wait, wait! We need you here!" Bill yelled.

Nick looked at me and ordered, "Step on it."

It was to no avail. Bill Batista and another supervisor quickly stood in front of my ambulance.

"They're blocking us," I said.

"Shit," Nick said, disappointed.

Nicholas Terranova, who was in charge of the medic school, had to be pried out of my ambulance, trying to get into the action.

Instead, Carl Mueller, who had made his way to the hospital from New Jersey, jumped into the passenger's seat, and we were off to the races.

As we drove down Seventh Avenue, the crowds cheered us. For

once it seemed as if the residents of Lower Manhattan would not be complaining of our noisy diesel engines keeping them up at night or our sirens and lights disturbing their sleep. No one was holding their ears as we screeched past them. Carl and I knew that it would be short-lived, but for the moment it was nice to know that they were on our side.

We flew toward Canal Street and saw that there were police barricades and uniformed men lining the streets. It did not look like we were going to get too far, but I was determined to get to the big show and so was Carl. Nothing was going to stop us from finding our friends and brothers. I was surprised to see Carl sitting in the tech seat and not putting up a fight about me driving. Carl pouts if he has to tech. He later hinted to me that he suffers from claustrophobia. It made sense because I noticed on several occasions that he gets red in the face and sweats profusely whenever he is in the back of the ambulance. At the moment, I think everyone was putting his or her neurosis aside.

"How long is this ride going to last?" Carl asked.

"Not long," I said, sensing that we would be stopped at any moment.

As we drove by the First Precinct on Varick Street and North Moore, there was a group of young men and women in green scrubs, interns and residents from St. Vincent's, making their way up to the front on foot. I pulled over the ambulance and yelled out of the window.

"Hey! Hop in."

"What are you doing?" Carl asked.

"Trust me," I replied.

The group of young doctors piled into the back and we were off again with lights and sirens blaring.

At the first checkpoint several police officers were directing us west. I opened the window and yelled out, "We got a bus full of doctors. We have to get them to the forward triage area." Carl just looked at me and smiled.

"The forward triage area? Where the hell is that?" he asked in a loud whisper.

"How the hell do I know? I'm making this up as I go."

The police officers waved us through as if we were admirals on a Navy base.

We drove downtown a couple of blocks, still on Varick Street. There was a young sergeant at the next checkpoint. It was Bobby Donnelly.

The Donnelly family lived down the street from my house when I lived on Staten Island. I knew the Donnellys for over twenty-five years. Jack, the Donnelly father, was in charge of plant supervision for the high school where I used to teach. He was a no-nonsense kind of guy. He was a retired cop who had been seriously injured in the line of duty. On a high-speed chase, he went crashing through the windshield on the passenger's side of his RMP (radio motor patrol car), which left him with a plate in his head and permanently disabled. He had a large family and three of his sons were police officers.

"Bobby, am I glad to see you. Where are your brothers?"

"They are both OK, but my sister Colleen was working in the Towers."

My heart sank. I taught most of the Donnelly children. Colleen was one of them. Days later I heard that she was safe and had made her way to her brother's precinct. She had the good sense to stay at the precinct house until he was contacted.

46

When the first plane hit, she was told to go back into the building, like so many others, as there was no chance of further threat. "Everything was under control," said building safety officers. Thankfully, Colleen was her father's daughter and didn't listen. She managed to get herself out and convinced others to go, as well.

The building safety officers were taking their orders from people who were supposedly much more informed. It's unfair to say that the safety officers were at fault. Safety officers were probably the last people to leave their posts, and almost all of them lost their lives.

"I'm sure that they got a lot of people out," Carl said, trying to reassure Bobby.

Bobby didn't answer, and waved us through.

We dropped the doctors off at a safe distance from the Towers. They headed towards West Street to find their fellow physicians. We continued south.

We made it to two blocks east of the Towers. Suddenly it felt like an atomic blast. It was 10:27 a.m. The first building to be hit, the North Tower of the World Trade Center, collapsed. We were at Ground Zero.

9
lost hero

After the North Tower fell I had no sense of time or space. My ears were ringing and my head was pounding. All I knew was that we headed as far south as we could in a direct line to where the Towers had been. It was like being in the middle of a snowstorm. The sky was dark and the air was filled with pulverized cement. What looked and had the consistency of volcanic ash covered our clothes, and lime dust filled our lungs. Carl and I had no masks and no helmets. We pulled up our shirts over our noses and headed out of the ambulance. We saw a lonely figure in the distance, a lost hero. He was a big hulk of a man wandering aimlessly and looking bewildered.

"What's up, brother?" Carl said.

"I can't find my truck. I can't find my crew," said the dazed man.

As we got face-to-face with the tired-looking figure, we saw that he was a firefighter who apparently got separated from his crew. He was one of the lucky ones who escaped from the North Tower before it fell. He must have started walking east and became disoriented. The man was obviously shell-shocked.

"We'll find them. But let's take a look at you, first," said Carl.

Carl led the firefighter into the back of the ambulance. I took a few steps further into the cloud and tried to gain my orientation, or at least find some daylight. I looked up, but saw nothing but darkness.

"My name is Mike," said the firefighter.

"My name is Carl."

"Hi, Carl."

Despite his idiosyncrasies, Carl Mueller is one of the kindest men I know. Although he sports a gruff appearance, which comes from a previous career as a police officer, he has one of the gentlest hearts that God has ever created.

Just as my eyes were about to shut from the blowing cement, I saw two more figures. It looked like they had federal badges, but it was hard to tell.

"How did you get down here?" said one of the men.

"We're paramedics from St. Vincent's."

"This area is secured. There are no more people here. They all high-tailed it to the river."

"You better check again. We got a fireman in the back of our bus."

"No shit?"

The other man quickly got on the radio.

"Sector three. One injured MOS found by EMS." An MOS is a member of service or uniformed personnel.

"Sector three, this is command. What the hell is EMS doing there? That area is supposed to be secured," Dispatch fired back.

"That's kind of a moot point. If they found somebody, you better send ESU to check the area again."

ESU is the Emergency Service Unit of the police department. They are police officers who are also EMTs or paramedics.

I suddenly heard Carl's voice coming from the back of the ambulance; "I think this guy's having an MI."

Sure as hell, the guy was having ST elevations in several EKG leads, indicating that he was having a myocardial infarction, otherwise known as a heart attack. This was in addition to coughing his brains out.

"Let's rock and roll," I said.

I drove east to West Broadway and headed north to St. Vincent's. Carl had a nonrebreather oxygen mask on the firefighter and was getting ready to start an IV line. Normally, we would take the time to work this guy up at the scene but this was not a normal day. Carl gave him an aspirin and a nitro-glycerine tablet en route. His blood pressure was still normal, but he wanted to get an IV line into him in case his blood pressure dropped from additional doses of nitro.

I called the dispatcher on the radio.

"Go St. Vincent's," the dispatcher replied.

"We have a forty-seven-year-old MOS, looks like he's having an inferior wall MI. He has ST elevations in leads two, three, and AVF (augmented voltage of the left foot leads). He's sinus tach at one-sixteen and he is normotensive. He's gotten an aspirin and nitro times one. He has difficulty breathing due to inhalation of cement dust and he has a productive cough. No known medical history, meds, or allergies."

"What is your ETA?"

"We are about two minutes out."

I heard a couple of more transmissions on the radio. "Good job, St. Vinny's," and "Godspeed." It must have been from other units in the field.

I thought to myself that it must have been a sorry state of affairs if we were getting kudos for bringing in one patient. There should be thousands of patients heading towards St. Vincent's. Hopefully they all made it to the river or at least to the triage center at Chelsea Piers.

We got to St. Vincent's in a matter of minutes. Everybody was cooperating and moving out of our way. A block away from the hospital, Carl yelled to me, "Frankie! Pull over!"

I immediately thought the worst. I figured the guy crapped out and Carl had to shock him. Whenever a patient needs to be shocked, the safest thing to do is pull the ambulance off the road so the medic does not accidentally shock himself.

I pulled over and saw what looked like a thousand hospital personnel in the distance waiting to pounce on our ambulance.

"Carl. What's the matter?"

"I can't get this damn line," he said.

I saw Carl desperately trying to start an IV. In normal circumstances it's pretty difficult to get a line in in a fast moving ambulance, but this guy was covered with dust and was probably dehydrated.

"Carl. Screw the line."

"I don't want us to look like asses when we pull up to the hospital."

"Carl. Not more than a hundred yards from us are about a thousand doctors and nurses who are dying to stick a needle in this guy's arm. Screw how we look!"

As our vehicle pulled into the ambulance bay, Nick, one of the paramedic supervisors, approach our vehicle. "As soon as you get your patient unloaded clear the ambulance bay," he said.

It looked as if the whole hospital came out to greet us. Doctors and nurses quickly pulled the firefighter out of the ambulance and rushed him into the ER.

I drove the ambulance a block away and parked it on Seventh Avenue near West Eleventh Street.

A pretty young doctor in a lab coat trotted up to my ambulance followed by Dr. Stephanie Wilkes.

"Am I glad to see you. Are you alright?" Stephanie asked as if I just came back from the dead.

"I'm fine."

"Did you happen to see Andrew?" the other doctor asked.

Realizing that she was the fiancée of Andrew Johns, I got a tremendous lump in my throat. Andrew must have bought the farm, I thought.

"I was east of the Towers. We were the only unit there. Five Willie, Andrew's unit, was west of us. I'm sure he's alright."

I saw her eyes fill up with tears.

"He'll be back. I promise."

She put her eyes down and walked slowly back to the hospital. Stephanie continued to look at me and I just shrugged my shoulders, not knowing if Andrew would ever come back. It was then that I saw Stephanie's eyes fill with tears. She gave me an uncomfortable smile, turned quickly and followed the other doctor back to the hospital, putting her arm around her as they both walked in silence.

I felt like a failure not being able to give her any words of consolation. I also felt terrible that Andrew was down at the Towers and I had no way to find him. That should have been me, I thought. "I pray to Christ that he's alright," I said to myself out loud.

Carl walked across the street from the hospital and hopped into the back of the ambulance.

"They want us to go to the staging area at Chelsea Piers. I'll finish cleaning the ambulance on our way over," he said.

10
chelsea piers

By the time we reached the Chelsea Piers, Carl had cleaned the back of our ambulance and made up the stretcher. There were dozens of ambulances lining West Street. Most of the vehicles were from New York hospitals and FDNY-EMS, with a few ambulances from neighboring New Jersey. I pulled up to the front of the line of ambulances in a vacant spot.

I noticed two other medics from St. Vincent's, Joe Moffitt and Desmond Engle, about ten vehicles behind us. I had seen them earlier when I arrived at the garage and I thought that by this time they would be in the thick of it. Instead, they sat in the long line; neither of them looked too happy about being there. Like everyone else they wanted to get into the action.

When I stopped the vehicle, Carl quickly jumped out of the back and lit a cigarette. I fished out a crumpled pack of cigarettes from my pants pocket and did the same. It was the first breather we had had since the whole thing started. We shook our heads in amazement of what just happened to us. It was a good release.

I glanced back and saw that the ambulance behind us was from St. Frances Cabrini Hospital. I recognized the EMT standing there and walked up to him. "Hi, Aaron. Thank God that you are alright."

Aaron was one of the EMTs who had taught my EMT class at Hatzolah Ambulance. Hatzolah was a volunteer ambulance corps in Brooklyn, mainly made up of orthodox Jews. They were a fairly large organization and were up at the front throughout the day, desperately trying to help. Aaron spoke with tears in his eyes.

"My partner was up at the Trades. I haven't heard from him yet."

"I'm sorry. I'm sure he got out."

His partner was Marc Sullins, an EMT from Cabrini Hospital, who went back into the building after taking patients to his ambulance. He was one of the missing.

Phil Generoso, a St. Vincent's paramedic, walked up to me followed by his fiancée Helen, who is also a paramedic, and who was his partner on that day. I saw Phil earlier that morning when he got off his shift on Three Victor, tour one. He was dressed in a Long Island College Hospital uniform, where he picks up extra tours.

"Hi, Papa," he said.

"Thank God you and Helen are alright. Where were you when they got hit?"

"We were sitting in our ambulance by the Brooklyn Bridge, eating breakfast, when we saw the plane hit. We went six-three [proceeding to the location] right away. Helen got on the radio and told central that a plane crashed into the Empire State Building!"

We both let out a nervous laugh.

"Thank God we cancelled choir practice this morning," I said.

"Where is Peter?"

"I don't know," I replied as I looked toward the Towers.

Just then I saw Kendra Camp out of the corner of my eye. She had met up with Phil and Helen and was now part of their crew. "Kendra!"

"Sorry I bugged out on you," she said, shaking her head as if embarrassed.

I didn't even acknowledge her statement. I knew that she had legitimate reasons for leaving me. "How are your kids?"

"They're fine. They're at home with my husband. Turns out that we couldn't leave the city even if we tried. The whole city is sealed off. No one in or out. I can't imagine what people at Vinny's think of me."

"The hell with what people think!"

As we talked there was a commotion up ahead. We headed back to our vehicles, looking to get on the road again. A middle-aged EMS lieutenant in a sweat-soaked uniform walked up to each bus and took our unit numbers. We were told to stand by and wait to be dispatched. After about ten minutes we realized that this was turning into a "clusterfuck," and we might be sitting there indefinitely. I looked at Carl and gave him a smile. I put on my lights and pulled out onto West Street. I glanced at my rearview mirror and saw the EMS lieutenant staring at our bus with a confused look on his face. Carl spoke up.

"Well, you gotta die of something."

"What is he going to do? Write us up?"

11
purgatory

We headed south again, not realizing that Phil, Helen and Kendra were not far behind us.

We passed each checkpoint and blasted our sirens and horn. The police officers manning the barricades just assumed that we had someplace to go. I learned this trick when I was in show business. That is how I'd audition without an appointment. *Always look like you belong someplace and no one will ever question you.*

We made it as far as BMCC, the Borough of Manhattan Community College, five blocks away from where the Trades once stood. Abruptly, we ran out of road.

A high-ranking EMS officer on the scene walked up to our vehicle, and I was sure that we were going to be reprimanded. I looked at him and said, "Here we are," and quickly started to check out my medical equipment. It was my best acting performance to date!

"Park your vehicle at a ninety-degree angle and stand by. Keep the engine running," the officer ordered matter-of-factly. Carl held in a laugh and shook his head.

We got out of our vehicle and it finally dawned on us what had happened. A cloud of smoke was where the Trades once stood and from the cloud we saw an endless line of men leaving the devastated area.

In the courtyard area of BMCC there were hundreds of firefighters sitting in silence, drinking water, some with their eyes closed, appearing to be in a total state of shock. Carl and I made our way through the sea of men, seeing if we could help anybody at all. We did a quick medical examination of those who would let us. We handed them bottles of water and sometimes poured the cool liquid over their heads and wounds. Our job was no longer search and rescue, but helping the men who had just come out of the belly of the beast. Our mission was not in hell but rather in purgatory.

We stood by our ambulance for a while and met up with Sal Ceriello. Sal was a handsome, good-natured young man of about twenty-five who was our classmate in medic school. He was a former marine and had just re-enlisted, this time in the Navy, two days before the crash.

Sal greeted us, "Hey guys!"

"How the hell did you get here?" asked Carl, obviously happy to see a familiar face.

"I was supposed to leave for boot camp this morning. I'm going to be a corpsman in the Navy. Everything got cancelled."

"Hang with us today," I said.

Sal got himself into the city from New Jersey and, by chance, happened to meet up with our ambulance. He became the third member of our crew that day.

"I'm not a New York City medic," he said, worried that he might be breaking some rules.

"Who gives a crap," I said, as Carl nodded in agreement, knowing full well that if the shit hit the fan, neither Carl, nor

I, nor anybody else was going to ask for his credentials.

"I'm going to take a walk. I've got a radio," I said, leaving the two of them to converse.

I walked a block south to view the destruction for myself. I still had the worst migraine of my life and there were no drugs for me to take. I guess I could have taken a handful of the baby aspirin that we kept onboard, but I was saving that for the patients.

I wandered over to the forward triage area at Stuyvesant High School. Luckily, all of the teenage students were evacuated safely. I ran into an ex–St. Vincent's paramedic, Deborah Silverman. When she worked at St. Vincent's, Deborah never gave me the time of day. She was a real cold broad. On that day she ran up to me, hugged me, and gave me a big kiss. I guess she was glad to see someone that she knew who was still alive.

In the hastily organized triage area I was surprised to see only a few patients, mostly uniformed personnel. I saw the doctors we had dropped off and many of the other residents and physician assistants from St. Vincent's. There were also dozens of medical students. This was a St. Vincent's show.

I looked at the horrible devastation in complete disbelief and total awe. How the hell did this happen? Why did they collapse? It looked like a bombed-out street in Europe during World War Two. I am a native New Yorker and I have lived and/or worked in New York City all of my life. I could not even make out where West Street once was because I was so disoriented.

I heard Carl's voice squawk over the radio: "Frankie, they want us to move our bus!"

I doubled back to the ambulance.

FDNY-EMS officers moved us back to another area closer to

North Moore Street. This time a very young lieutenant addressed our small group of EMTs and our lone paramedic unit.

"I want you to keep your vehicles parked at a ninety-degree angle and shut the engines off. The people up ahead will bring the patients to us," he ordered. "We want you to conserve fuel. We don't know if there will be any more fuel available to us."

Carl spoke up. "What happens if we can't start the vehicles? Wouldn't it be better to just keep them running?"

Carl's suggestion was falling on deaf ears. A few minutes later, Carl gloated when an ambulance had to be jump-started.

I was trying to get a call through on my cell phone to my family, but there was no cellular service. I thought it was a good idea not to continue, since my battery was almost dead and I did not want to tie up the cells with unnecessary chatter in case there was some poor bastard under the rubble trying to get some help. "Where the hell is Peter?" I asked. Carl just gave me a serious look.

We did a double take when we saw an FDNY ambulance pass by with two paramedics from St. Vincent's. I shouted to Carl, "Hey, look at that ambulance!"

Apparently two of our medics had commandeered an abandoned ambulance and were in the process of transporting patients. One of the medics smiled slyly at me and the other was chuckling, proud of his ingenuity. I shook my head and tipped my baseball cap as they passed by. It suddenly dawned on me that the crew of the abandoned ambulance might have been inside the Towers when they crashed. I just hoped the reason that the rig was abandoned was that the original crew was still alive and had to make a run for it.

Our brief respite was broken when a middle-aged man in a filthy uniform was wheeled up to one of the EMT vehicles.

"What's the problem?" Carl inquired of the EMTs who seemed confused about how to treat him.

"This FDNY officer is having difficulty seeing," said the young EMS lieutenant who was also an EMT.

Being the only paramedics in the area, Carl and I started to check him out. Basically, we were in charge of patient care.

"Let's take a look," I said while gently trying to open his tightly shut eyes.

The patient was an FDNY chief. He had dust and crud caking his eyes.

"Let's get him on our stretcher," Carl commanded the others.

"It doesn't hurt. Just give me some drops and let me get back to the front," the chief requested.

"First, we want to wash your eyes out with saline, sir," I said while trying to examine his eyes.

"Screw that. My men are up there," the chief argued.

"It's OK, Chief. We'll take care of it," said a young firefighter who held the hand of his commander tightly.

Months later I found out that our patient was Battalion Commander Richard Picciotto, who had been trapped in a stairwell when Tower One collapsed. He lived to write about his harrowing escape in his book *Last Man Down*.

"Why don't you give him some proparacaine drops?" suggested the young EMS lieutenant.

"We want to irrigate his eyes first," explained Carl.

"Besides, proparacaine's for pain and deadens the eyes. It'll make him feel like he has two giant meatballs in his head," I added.

"Let's take him to Vinny's," Carl said.

Carl and the others quickly got Chief Picciotto onto our stretcher, despite his protests, and began to irrigate his eyes with bottles of saline. I spiked an IV bag and street-rigged a line cut from a nasal cannula, a plastic tubing with a double opening designed to administer oxygen via both nostrils. It provided irrigation to both of his eyes at the same time. Since we did not know the nature of the substance that was in his eyes, and Chief Picciotto claimed that he was not in pain, we held off on the proparacaine drops.

I drove to St. Vincent's while Carl squeezed a second bag of saline en route.

Again we were met by a storm of health care workers eager to help.

12
ground zero

A block away from the hospital, Carl and I were cleaning up the back of our ambulance when an attractive young woman with dark brown hair walked up to us and started speaking.

"I am from the *Daily News*. If you're going back there, could you take me with you?"

Carl said, "That's a restricted area. We don't even know if they will let us back down there."

She then started asking us some questions. Carl spoke eloquently about what was going on and she asked me some questions as well.

I do not take credit for coining the phrase, but during the course of the interview I stated that it looked like "ground zero" after a nuclear attack.

She responded, "Ground Zero. I like that," as she wrote down my comment.

"Any word about Peter?" I asked Carl after the reporter left our area.

"Not yet. Sorry," responded Carl.

"What about our crews?"

"They're all safe. They got them working light duty at the hospital. They want to know if we want some R and R."

"What for? We didn't do anything yet."

Somehow Andrew Johns made it back to the hospital alive. Happily, I saw Andrew and his fiancée talking to each other and smiling. They kept kissing each other and looking tenderly into one another's eyes. I felt a moment of sadness that there was no one in my life who I believed cared for me that way or looked at me in that way anymore.

My trance was broken when Carl came back to the ambulance. I looked at him and said, "Let's go, sweetheart!"

He looked at me as if I had three heads. "When did you change teams?" he asked.

"Believe me, you will be the first one to know."

"Let's get going before they keep us in the rear!" Carl ordered.

"Screw Chelsea Piers! That's a hurry up and wait area," I said.

We headed back to the North Moore Street forward staging area. With the other four crews reassigned to 911 and hospital duties, we would be the only St. Vincent's unit up at the front.

We no sooner got our ambulance parked on North Moore Street than a group of New York's bravest wheeled a firefighter to our vehicle. He was having a heart attack. This time we treated him on scene, and Carl had no problem getting in the IV line.

We were greeted by smiling faces at the hospital. Nick said, "Are you guys back again?" As if we were the only ambulance bringing in patients. Actually, more than six hundred patients were treated at St. Vincent's that day. All of them were treated gratis. Most of the uniformed personnel had minor injuries and eye irritations. The number of police and firefighters who were treated is unknown, since they refused to be documented. They just wanted to get fixed up and go back into action. Interns and residents worked frantically to pour saline solution into their eyes and to clean and take care of their wounds.

By the time we brought our newest patient into the ER and cleaned up our bus, it was around noon and the hospital was crowded with generous New Yorkers eager to donate blood, donate food, or volunteer in any way possible. Off-duty medics were pouring into the city ready to go to work. The medic supervisors again asked Carl and me if we needed relief. After all, we had gone for two days without sleep, but we declined. We were just fine.

"Back to North Moore Street?" I asked Carl, with a new surge of energy.

"I don't want to go back to the forward staging area and be under the command of some baby-faced kid who doesn't know what the fuck he's doing!" Carl snapped.

He was right. Our young lieutenant on North Moore was making it up as he was going along, probably because there was no real central command. Every officer in the field was on their own. We started to slowly realize that *everyone* was on their own.

Carl and I headed towards the front again, but first we stopped at the ambulance garage to pick up supplies and try to find a couple of helmets.

When we arrived at the garage, I found out that Paramedic Marco Farina, whom I had left in charge, had abandoned it. Joe Moffit and Desmond Engle were now in charge of the official walking wounded triage center, unofficially dubbed "the Oasis."

"He met up with some of his volunteer fireman buddies from Long Island and decided to be a high-profile hero," said Desmond. "He's off digging in the Pile."

"We don't mind doing this job. It beats the hell out of waiting around at Chelsea Piers," said Joe.

Marco, like most of us, wanted to do something courageous. His digging at the Pile earned him the name of "Powder," since he was covered with dust upon his return. This derogatory nickname became a term of endearment that was even appreciated by Marco in the months that followed. Everyone was looking to earn a medal of honor and Powder was his.

Carl and I scrounged up a couple of helmets, but there were no supplies to be found. In the early minutes of the crash other units stockpiled their ambulances, not realizing there would be anybody else looking for supplies.

Sensing our frustration Joe said, "I told those guys not to take all the supplies."

"If all hell breaks loose we're screwed," I said.

"Welcome to nine-eleven," said Desmond.

Carl and I wormed our way up to the front line, bypassing North Moore Street and other check points. The police were restricting the flow of vehicles up to the front.

As we monitored the radio, Central Dispatch was assigning unit numbers to every ambulance in the city. All additional crews were known as enhancement units.

"St. Vincent's vehicle number seventeen-fifty-one you are now Fifty-one William, tour two," the dispatcher announced, which was all right by us since our vehicle, seventeen-fifty-one, was used for Five William, tour one. It was easy to remember and a good set of numbers.

We posted ourselves as close to the front line as possible as a call came over Central Dispatch.

"Any ALS unit in the vicinity of One World Trade Center report to the sector commander."

"Fifty-one William, put us Sixty-three," I replied. The dispatcher acknowledged our transmission.

"Fifty-one William, eighty-eight," I said into the radio, announcing our arrival at Ground Zero.

When we arrived, we saw what it was really all about. Thousands of firefighters and police were huddled together as if in a landing craft on D-Day, ready to deploy on the beaches at Normandy. We stood shoulder to shoulder with our brothers, smelling their sweat and feeling their body heat. All of the men's faces looked old, although many were clearly in their twenties. We were all old men that hot day in September.

We walked up to a lone Cornell Medical Center BLS unit manned by two EMTs and we helped load the body of Peter J. Ganci, Jr., twenty-eighth chief of the Fire Department, or what was left of the brave soul, onto their ambulance for transport to the morgue. Even though the man was clearly deceased, the reason Central called for paramedics was that those in command wanted to make sure nothing else could be done for their beloved chief.

"He really gone?" A firefighter in his twenties asked with tears filling his eyes.

"I'm sorry," I said. "I'm truly sorry."

A young Catholic chaplain in a cassock and dirty stole administered last rites. Carl made the sign of the cross and blessed himself, as did many of the men in our immediate vicinity.

Earlier that day Chief Ganci had escaped death when the

South Tower collapsed.

Ganci then set up his command post near the North Tower and continued to supervise rescue efforts. When it was feared that the North Tower might also collapse, he ordered all personnel out of the area, including his personal staff. Like a captain of a ship, he refused to leave the men that were still in the North Tower who had not returned from their mission. When the North Tower collapsed, Chief Ganci gave his life, refusing to leave his post.

Knowing his exact last known whereabouts made it easier for his staff to search and find what was left of their fallen commander.

"EMS wants a city unit," said a FDNY captain.

Smoke and heat were pouring out of the smoldering ashes of the Towers and buildings burned all around us. While we stood there awaiting orders and holding vigil with our brothers, we were told to evacuate the area because the Millennium Hotel, which was directly east of us, was about to collapse.

Carl and I got back into our vehicle which was now at the end of the line, since the other vehicles that had filed behind us were now in front of us. That single moment was the only time that I felt any kind of panic. The minutes slowly passed as we sat there waiting to leave.

Carl smoked cigarette after cigarette. I started to get angry and wanted to jump out and search through the Pile. If I were to die I wanted to die on sanctified ground. Not many men get to pick the time, the place, and the form of their death. I wanted to die trying to save lives rather than in a traffic jam. After what seemed like an eternity we started to move.

We were deployed several blocks away from the crash site, facing the tallest remaining tower, building Number Seven of the World Trade Center complex, forty-seven stories high, which stood between the North and South Towers. Earlier, parts of the Twin Towers had crashed into building Seven and set it ablaze. Diesel fuel stored for emergency generator use and jet fuel from the original crash were causing it to burn out of control. Our day had just begun.

13
the safe zone

The tallest remaining tower was engulfed in flames. A lone FDNY ladder company was dousing the building with water in what looked like a futile attempt to contain the fire. Other firefighters and police officers were in the vicinity of Warren Street, a block south of Chambers Street, standing ready to direct any traffic that happened to wander into the area.

"Turn your ambulances around and face south," one EMS officer ordered over a portable public address system.

The strategy was to turn our ambulances in the right direction in case we had to rush into the hot zone when casualties were finally found.

We received the same order as before: "Turn off your motors. You need to conserve fuel!" Carl rolled his eyes and shook his head vigorously.

As the hours passed, we monitored the Manhattan frequencies. There was all kinds of chatter including reports of finding casualties, but these were unsubstantiated. BEMS and FDNY officers occasionally came into the area to rebrief us.

We could feel the air get hotter and more humid as the fire company poured water on the burning building. I reported to my commanders back at St. Vincent's via Nextel Direct Connect.

"This is Fifty-one William. Rella and Mueller. We're standing by at Greenwich and Chambers."

Nextels were the only communications that were reliable on the eleventh. That was because central cellular antennas had been mounted on the Twin Towers. Nextel uses a two-way communication system similar to a walkie-talkie, and does not need a central antenna as cellular phones do.

"Do you want relief, guys?" a familiar voice asked.

"Negative, Nick. We're not leaving. We're alright."

Carl and I both felt that we had not done anything yet. We were not going back to the rear area. Most of the St. Vincent's paramedic staff had reported to the hospital and they wanted to get their crack at the front lines, but there was no way that Carl and I would voluntarily leave.

"Nick. Any word about Pete Castellano?"

"Pete's OK. He's working the triage center at the garage. He's been worried about you."

"Thank God!" I said to Carl, as a wave of relief spread across my body. I guess it was endorphins, because I suddenly felt my headache subside. "OK, Nick. Send him my regards. Tell him I'm going to kick his ass next time I see him for not calling me."

"He told me to give you the same message."

Peter had made his way home without hearing about the initial crash. When he got there his wife pleaded with him not to go back into the city. He momentarily sat on his couch and stared at the TV, confused and in disbelief. Being the marine that he is, he knew his duty and immediately left for Manhattan once he realized what was going on. Unfortunately, the city was already sealed off and he had a hell of a time getting back in.

Upon arriving, Peter was put in charge of the triage area at the ambulance garage and treated the walking wounded. He later relieved Gary Chester and Esteban Guerrero on Three Victor, tour two. He was eventually partnered up with Ned Edwards, who was reassigned to regular 911 duties.

Sometime in the afternoon, we decided that waiting this close to building Number Seven could possibly be another disaster in the making for the ambulance crews. Our vehicles had no way out if the building came toppling down. We were told by our superiors that it would not fall, but at that point I did not trust their judgment. I turned my ambulance around and faced it north, in the opposite direction of building Number Seven, in case we had to make a run for our lives. Carl and I went around to the other ambulance crews and made them do the same. We also told them to turn on their engines and keep them running. We could always turn our ambulances around again if we had to head towards Ground Zero.

We got into a heated argument with one of the FDNY-EMS crews, because they did not want to disobey orders from their officers.

"Guys, just turn your goddamn bus around!" I said.

"Our captain told us to stand by in this direction. Maybe we should listen to them, Rella!" said an FDNY EMT sarcastically, reading the name tag on my shirt.

"Don't you guys get it? It's been hours since we've seen an officer. For all practical purposes we're on our own."

"You guys can't order us around just because you're paramedics. You're not even FDNY. Besides, I don't want to get written up."

"It's not an order, brother. Just think of it as friendly advice," Carl said.

Carl and I looked at each other as if we were about to use more physical means of persuasion, but the EMT's partner quietly got into the ambulance and turned the vehicle around.

"What the hell are you doing?" the EMT yelled to his partner.

"Following friendly advice," the other man said.

14
the third tower

At around 5:20 p.m., building Number Seven collapsed. There was no official order to take cover, or an order to evacuate.

I heard that the building was falling from people screaming outside of my ambulance. I put my head down and braced for the worst. I literally saw my life pass in front of me. I saw my new bicycle at Christmas, the first time I kissed a girl, the birth of my two beautiful daughters, how stunning Tammy looked on our wedding day, my mother's face, baptizing my own son's lifeless body, and also every moment of failure that I regretted in my life. Everything I was ever sorry for doing or not doing. I knew my life was over and there were so many things that I was going to miss.

I just asked God for courage and spoke a final prayer out loud. It was not a prayer for forgiveness. I believed that God already knew I was sorry for my sins and, in his mercy, I hoped he forgave me. Instead it was the prayer of St. Dismas, the good thief, who was crucified at the cross with Jesus: "Remember me, Lord, when You come into Your Kingdom."

I hoped the next face I would see would be that of my grandmother Rose, leading me to and defending me at my final judgment. It was then that I heard someone yell to evacuate the ambulance and take cover. It was probably Carl.

The high-pitched squeal of bending steel was followed by what sounded like a nuclear bomb headed in our direction. The ground shook like an earthquake. I jumped out and went to the front of the ambulance to take cover. Carl and Sal Ceriello were trying to squeeze under the front bumper to no avail. Sal was covering Carl's top half while I jumped on Carl's lower half.

"For Chrissakes, Carl, get your ass down," I yelled as we all pressed our bodies against each other, forcefully into the ground.

We were too close to the building and started to get pelted with debris. This was it. We were dead and we knew it. The only comfort was that we were going to die with our brothers. It was then that I heard Carl yell to me to get into the bus. I looked up and somehow he and Sal were already in the ambulance and waving at me to get in. I jumped into the driver's seat and searched quickly for my keys. They were already in the ignition. I had inadvertently left them there. Thank God that the ambulance was still running.

I took off, blasting my horn and hitting the siren. We slowed down, yelling out the window at the other crews to follow us. We saw them get into their vehicles and file behind us one by one, as if awaking from a deep sleep . We drove a couple of blocks north to safety. None of the dozen or so crews were injured.

The FDNY crew that argued with us earlier ran up to our bus.

"Thank you. Thank you," they said over and over to Carl and me as they hugged us with tears in their eyes.

We drove down to the original staging area, this time nearer to Warren Street, and parked our vehicle facing the fallen building to the south. It would be impossible to drive up to the collapsed building, so we gathered our medical bags and proceeded on foot. We were half-crazed after what had just happened, and we were not waiting around for any more orders.

"Sal, you stay with the bus," I yelled as Carl and I continued to walk south.

A bunch of EMTs got the same idea but they stopped short of the ensuing dust cloud. Carl and I walked right past them as smoke and powdered cement engulfed us. We found some surgical masks in our medical bag and put them over our faces and waded through the debris and smoke. As we continued to walk into the dust cloud we passed some firefighters and police officers.

"Are you guys hurt?" Carl asked.

"No, we're alright."

"Any injuries up ahead? Are there any men down there?" I asked.

"We don't know," the shaken men answered.

We asked everyone we met if there were any injuries, but nobody quite knew. Carl and I made it to within a half a block from where building Number Seven once stood, but the heat was no longer bearable. Our skin was getting incredibly hot and the hair on our arms started to singe. We had no scott packs (air tanks) or protective gear. All we had were paper dust masks and our cotton summer uniforms to protect us.

Thankfully, there were no injuries. When we were sure of this, we thought it best to get out of the hot zone and stand by our ambulance and figure out what to do next. As we began to exit from the cloud, the EMTs approached us. They were adhering to the cardinal rule of EMS, which is "scene safety."

"When we didn't see you come out right away we decided to

come in after you," said the EMT who had refused to turn his ambulance around.

"Thanks, brother. There are no casualties. Let's all get the hell out of here before we pass out," I said coughing and hacking. They all followed us out.

As we walked towards our vehicles, a platoon of ESU police marched into the cloud in full regalia and facemasks. If there were casualties to be found, any that we might have missed, they would be the ones to get the job done.

Carl and I went back to our ambulance and tried to clean up a bit. Sal was there guarding it, as I had requested.

"The old girl is looking pretty shabby," I remarked to Sal, deliberately pointing in Carl's direction.

"Who, Carl?" asked Sal, slightly shocked at my remark.

"No, the ambulance," I said with a straight face, as Carl looked at me and shook his head, smirking.

Vehicle 1751 was still purring away with her overworked diesel engine.

15
dusk, 9/11

Dusk set in, and there were no Towers to light the night skies. Power was lost or shut down in a large part of Lower Manhattan, and it was as if a curtain had been draped over the entire area. The air was thick with dust.

As night finally fell, caravans of trucks went charging past us, mostly units from out of town that had just arrived, hoping to get into the action and do some good. Vehicles from New Jersey and Long Island were carrying special units such as K-9s and crime-scene detachments. They kicked up an enormous amount of dust, most of it lodging in our eyes and filling our lungs.

Carl and I snidely swear that because we are both smokers we did not develop pulmonary problems. Our lungs were already coated with nicotine and that served as a protective covering. Both of us had nasty coughs, which still bother us today, as well as chronic eye irritation.

With all these reserve units pouring into the area it looked as if it was gearing up to be a pissing match. We began to see a barrage of conflicting orders from commanders jockeying for control of the scene. I am sure that they had good intentions, but they did not realize that most of us had almost been killed more than once that day.

They barked out their orders.

"Move your vehicles ten feet forward!"

"Move your vehicles ten feet back!"

"Turn off your engines!"

"Turn on your engines!"

It was madness!

Carl and I finally got a hold of some saline for our eyes that the Salvation Army workers had brought up to the front in cases. The cool liquid provided minimal relief. It actually made matters worse. The grit that had been annoying our eyeballs and contact lenses became mud when it mixed with the fluid.

"Oh, that makes everything much better. Now I can't see anything," Carl said, as his contact lenses became more hazed over.

We waited to hear any word about what was going on. The minutes and hours passed and there were still no orders from Central Dispatch. The chaos that had cluttered the airways had been replaced with a steady narrative of designator numbers for the new units that poured into the city. Central Dispatch was spewing high numbers like Sixty Victor and Ninety Tom. All of these units waited anxiously for something to do and somewhere to go.

As we sat there in the dark and the filth, triage and treatment areas were being set up all over the city. By chance, Madison Square Garden at Thirty-fourth Street was hosting a convention of surgeons that day. The visiting doctors quickly moved into action and set up a triage center there, replacing Chelsea Piers on Twenty-third Street. The Chelsea Piers now were being used strictly for a staging area, and hundreds of ambulances kept vigil there. Huge morgue areas were being set up at both Bellevue Hospital on First Avenue and at the Meadowlands Sports Complex in New Jersey. Retired police officers and

firefighters were being called up to active service to keep the peace
and sort out the honored dead.

Sal Ceriello had to leave our crew. He had been with us
throughout the day, leaving our ambulance occasionally to help
other crews and give assistance to the Salvation Army workers
in the area. He brought food to the ambulance crews and to other
emergency workers. Sal received a call from his recruiter that he
was to report to Fort Hamilton Army Post in Brooklyn. He
was going to be immediately sent to basic training now that we
were in a state of war. Carl and I said our goodbyes and carried
on with our work, wondering if we would ever see Sal again.

Late that night, we heard a call over the radio for a paramedic
unit. The injuries to the rescue workers began. We were only
blocks away, but it was difficult to get through to Central
Dispatch. They were ordering a unit from the Chelsea Piers to
take the call. By this time our whereabouts were pretty much
unknown to both our supervisors and the EMS command.

After our third attempt to contact Central Dispatch, we
received a reply.

"Fifty-one Willie, proceed."

I got on the onboard radio, bypassing Carl's handheld.

"Fifty-one Willie. We are a block from the Trade Center, let
us pick up that call, Central."

There was no response, so I repeated my transmission.
Still nothing.

The politics had begun. Little did we know that the voluntary
hospitals, and in particular St. Vincent's, were getting the
majority of the publicity. The press was making the city hospitals
and the Bureau of Emergency Medical Services (BEMS) look

as if they were not even involved. This was not done purposely; it was just the way the news was presented. St. Vincent's Hospital was the closest trauma center to the Trade Center. Even the FDNY-EMT units were taking the majority of the patients to St. Vincent's. At the time, there was no fast way to Bellevue Hospital, which was run by the city. Bellevue is at First Avenue and Twenty-seventh Street, the quick route to which was south of the Trade Center by way of the FDR drive. But that was blocked. You could travel north from our position, but you would pass St. Vincent's, Cabrini, NYU Downtown, and Beth Israel hospitals on your way.

It seemed that Central Dispatch was trying to get an FDNY-EMS unit down to the patient.

"Any municipal paramedic units in the area?" inquired the dispatcher, ignoring my previous transmissions.

BEMS, like everyone else, was trying to get into the action and, unfortunately, into the press.

I repeated my transmission one last time. Central Dispatch finally answered us.

"Stand by, Fifty-one William. Fifty-one Victor proceed to the location."

Now Carl was as pissed as I was.

"That's bullshit. It's a block away. They're keeping a patient waiting! Let's just go," he said.

Much to our surprise, as we entered the disaster site the patient was already being treated. A lone BLS unit from Long Island had "buffed" the job and was not going to tell Dispatch until they were on their way to St. Vincent's.

"Can you guys tell us how to get to Saint Vincent's?" one of the first aiders asked innocently.

Carl and I shook our heads and looked at one another in amazement. I almost started to laugh.

Near where we had stopped our vehicle we came upon a small gathering of ambulances and a couple of EMS officers who happened to be Chief McCracken and Deputy Chief McFarland. With his dust-caked eyes and lack of sleep Carl did not comprehend that the four stars on McCracken's collar meant that he was chief of all EMS. He looked squarely at McCracken and spoke: "Is there a supervisor here? We can't just be standing around here doing nothing."

McCracken looked directly at me and questioned, "Are you his partner?"

"Yes, sir," I replied, knowing that the stars on his collar did not mean that he was the Texaco man.

"What's wrong with him?" he asked in a commanding manner. I just covered my eyes with my hands and shook my head.

Before Carl could speak again, I put my index finger over my lips, gesturing at Carl not to talk. Carl looked at me with a confused look.

"I'll explain it to you later," I whispered loudly.

Deputy Chief McFarland, a young-looking man in his forties whom I remembered seeing with the body of Chief Ganci earlier that day, spoke to our group:

"You two paramedics and the rest of you report to the forward command center. I'll show you how to get there."

16

forward command center

The forward command center was set up in the American Express building, which was right next to where the Twin Towers once stood.

I snaked our ambulance around the debris and barely passable roadways. Carl and I exited our vehicle, pushing our stretcher up to the building. We had our cardiac monitor and medical bags on top of the stretcher.

The AMEX building was one big shit hole. Windows were blown out and debris was everywhere. A couple of doctors from St. Vincent's quickly walked up to us.

"Did you bring us any supplies?"

We looked at them, puzzled for a moment, and shook our heads, no.

"Can we at least have your tube kit in case we get any patients?"

This was a sorry place. Only two doctors and not a bit of gear. Just two anxious-looking men in scrubs who were probably conscripted from the rear area.

"Sorry, Doc. We are the only medic unit up here and we have to hang on to what we've got. When we get back to Vinny's we'll have another unit send you some stuff."

An EMS officer told us to line up our stretchers next to a half-dozen other units in the lobby and stand by.

After we set our gear down, I walked solemnly towards the east window and saw the devastation from another angle. Someone had hung an American flag in one of the blown out windows on the inside of the building. It was superimposed against the night sky with the rubble outside highlighted by bright emergency lights.

By this time a crane was pulling some vehicles from the Pile.

"Nothing survived the collapses," Carl said, as he joined me in looking out the window.

"I agree, brother."

"If anybody's still alive they're probably trapped in a pocket and would have to be fished out."

Carl and I went back to our stretcher and listened to a group of EMTs taking about the day's events. One of the crews said that they did dig some poor soul out late into the night.

"The guy was so crazed he probably would never be right in the head again."

We also heard other incredible rescue stories as the night passed.

"Did you hear that one guy rode the wave from the ninety-first floor as the building collapsed and had only a couple of broken bones to show for it?" said another EMT.

The most curious story was that the Towers collapsed because there were explosives strategically placed on every floor.

"There was explosion after explosion as the Towers crashed. Not only that, there were dozens of cars lined up around the Towers, and they exploded one after another at the precise moment that the planes hit the buildings. It was a coordinated attack," said an older EMT.

You had to take these stories with a grain of salt. Rumors and tall tales abounded.

The silence was broken when a cocky EMS lieutenant who was also an EMT stepped up to talk to us. In FDNY-EMS, officers can be either EMTs or paramedics. Their rank has nothing to do with their medical training. We had seen this lieutenant earlier as he sat among the other FDNY-EMT crews and held court. It looked as if BEMS was turning this into an FDNY show and we were unwelcome visitors.

"Dump your gear and your mattress. Follow me with your stretcher," the EMS lieutenant ordered.

Carl and I looked at each other slightly confused and slightly annoyed. We passed Deputy Chief McFarland, who was standing by a huge desk talking to an FDNY paramedic, as we wheeled our stretcher through the lobby and out into the night air.

The young lieutenant led us to a truck.

"You see those boxes? Load them on your stretcher," he ordered.

Carl and I complied and loaded as many boxes as possible onto our empty stretcher. He pointed us in the direction of the Pile and told us to dump our load at the edge of the pit.

We made quite a few trips and when the last box was loaded we realized that we were the only crew that was doing this manual labor.

When we were finished Carl asked, "What's in the boxes?"

"Body bags," he said.

When we saw him again holding court with his FDNY–EMT buddies and laughing, Carl and I were livid. Our blood pressure skyrocketed.

"I got the paramedics to do the shit work for a change," we heard him say.

Carl and I walked up to him and I said, "You know Lieutenant, we don't mind doing grunt work, if everybody is doing it with us."

Carl chimed in, "It seems that we're the only paramedic unit up here and you could make better use of our training."

Just then, we were interrupted by the FDNY medic who had been talking to the deputy chief earlier. He was white as a ghost as he spoke to us.

"I think the chief is having an MI."

We quickly grabbed our gear and ran over to the deputy chief. Sure as shit, McFarland was having a heart attack. The monitor was showing ST elevations in most of the leads. We quickly started a line on him and gave him some oxygen. We administered aspirin and nitroglycerin and loaded him onto the ambulance.

As a courtesy, and because he looked like he was genuinely concerned about McFarland, I asked the FDNY medic, "Do you want to take over the call?"

He looked at us and said, "No, you guys know what you're doing. You're Vinny's medics."

The FDNY medic hopped on the back of the bus and I started walking to the driver's side door. Carl stopped me.

"Let me drive."

"No way, I've been driving all day. You're teching."

Carl had this panicked look on his face. "Let me drive, please! This will be the only opportunity I get to drive. They're going to put us out of service when we get back."

"What's the big deal about driving?" I asked.

Carl just looked at me. I saw that he was clearly upset, although I did not really know the reason. I had been driving all day long. What was his sudden urge to drive? Did he finally reach his breaking point or did his claustrophobia increase when there was another person in the back of the ambulance?

All I really was sure of was that Carl looked as if all of the blood was drained from his face. Carl was a brave man and a competent medic, both of which he proved that day.

I did not wait for Carl to answer my last question. I just handed him the keys and walked to the back.

When we got to the checkpoint a hundred yards away from where we were parked, a crowd formed at the back of the ambulance. Apparently word had spread quickly that McFarland was having a heart attack. The ambulance door opened and a tall older man who was a high-ranking EMS officer started to speak. He completely ignored me and talked to the FDNY paramedic seated on the bench.

"You're taking him to Bellevue, right?"

The FDNY paramedic said nothing and glanced at me with wide eyes. I spoke right up. "That's a negative, sir, we are going to St. Vinny's."

"Who are you?"

"I am the paramedic in charge."

"He's going to Bellevue, son."

Noticing that he was wearing the patch of an EMT and not a paramedic I felt my blood pressure rise.

"I don't even know if there is a road open to Bellevue. I know there is one open to Vinny's."

"We'll open one for you. Just tell your driver to follow the police cars."

"No. Why don't you tell the police cars to follow my ambulance, because I already told the paramedic in the front to drive to Vinny's, sir."

"I am a division chief of EMS and you will go where I tell you to go, son."

"You have a patch that says *EMT* on your shoulder. I have a patch that says *paramedic* on mine, and you will get off my bus."

As I slammed the door in his face, he started to scream at me and told me he was going to put me on report. I couldn't really care since my main concern was to get McFarland to the closest hospital in the shortest amount of time.

I saw Carl in the front of the ambulance, looking as if he was trying to crawl under the steering wheel. He appeared more disturbed at my conversation with the division chief than he did when the building fell on him.

The crowd of FDNY personnel outside the ambulance looked through the window in disbelief, and the FDNY paramedic stared at me in the same way. I just shrugged my shoulders and continued to treat my patient. McFarland smiled at me and said, "I think you handled that diplomatically."

As we drove to the hospital, McFarland's pain started to increase, as did his EKG elevations, indicating that he had a real chance of going south or, in any case, of winding up with a transmural MI (a heart attack involving the entire muscle of the heart). If it got any worse he would lose significant cardiac tissue that would never regenerate. The prognosis would be that this young man would be virtually a cripple or, at best, would need a heart transplant.

Throughout the trip, McFarland showed true courage and didn't once openly complain about the pain that, from personal experience, I knew he was having.

I think I tried to call for orders, but I am not sure. I say that because if I did not call for orders, I would lose my paramedic card. You can give most drugs on standing orders, but you cannot give narcotics without an order from a doctor. In any case, I do remember drawing up five milligrams of morphine and giving the chief the dose. It pretty much stopped the pain of the MI in its tracks. With the additional doses of nitroglycerin, I think it did the trick. By the time we got him to St. Vincent's he was in pretty good shape. I heard later that he was released without any major damage and he returned to work shortly thereafter.

We quickly delivered Deputy Chief McFarland to the ER staff, parked the ambulance across the street, and speedily started cleaning up the ambulance.

"Let's get away before anybody notices us," Carl whispered loudly.

"If we worked for two days without sleep, we can work another two," I said.

Our supervisors were on to us immediately. All three of them came out to the bus, accompanied by two police officers.

They expressed their gratitude for a job well done and for the long hours we worked. "You guys did a great job," said Bill Batista.

"You guys are officially out of service," said Gabe Abrams.

"We're OK. Really," I said.

"We're going back to the forward command center," Carl said.

"By the way, guys, if you try to go back into service we're going to have you arrested," Nick said as he and the others gave us a big smile. "Go get some rest."

Carl and I tried to put up an argument, but it was to no avail. There were police officers on either side of the vehicle and the replacement crew was already in the back of our ambulance, restocking, as we continued arguing our point.

We were finally out of service for the day at about 1:30 a.m. on the morning of September 12.

17
the land of the free

Before we were sent to a hotel for a good night's sleep, I walked across the street to the local newsstand to pick up a pack of cigarettes. The pack that Carl gave me earlier that morning was long gone and I wanted to stock up for the days ahead. I thought we would be back at the front soon and I did not want to be without a nicotine fix.

As I waded through the crowd of onlookers, people were holding out cups of Starbucks coffee, sandwiches, and goody bags. Where did all these people come from? I wondered.

I entered the small store and was taken aback at first. The Middle-Eastern storekeeper, who I saw just about every day, started to make me feel uneasy while I waited in line. Why was he different to me today? Why was I looking at him as if he was the enemy? I started to feel ashamed of myself for wanting to hate him.

My shame was quickly replaced by anger when the two young men ahead of me on line started to harass him and call him names. I immediately changed moods and started to speak in his defense.

"Who the hell are you?" I asked.

The men reeled around and spoke.

"What's your problem?" one of them said.

"My problem is that you are bothering this guy."

"Why are you defending him?" the other guy asked.

"Because he is an American just like you, asshole."

"Why don't you mind your own fucking business?" the first guy said.

"This city is my business," I said, and then, "OK. You have a choice. You can either walk through that door or I can throw you through it."

They both looked at me in silence and saw that I wasn't kidding. They left, muttering to themselves.

I looked at the man behind the counter and said, "I'm sorry those guys were bothering you."

He started getting very excited. "Anything you want, you take, my friend. Thank you very much. Thank you very much," he repeated over and over again. I really started feeling like a heel because of my initial reaction.

To this day, whenever any hospital personnel or I go into that store, he practically gives his merchandise away. I was one step away from being a prejudiced jerk that somebody would want to throw through a door. I thank God that my mother did not bring me up that way. It made me realize that all Americans have a right to be here, including those who might look like the enemy.

18
working for peanuts

After being taken out of service in the early hours of the morning on September 12, a group of medics waited to be transported to temporary sleeping quarters. For the medics of St. Vincent's Hospital that meant the Hyatt Regency Hotel in midtown Manhattan.

We had it better than most. Instead of cots at an armory or some fleabag hotel or, worse yet, our filthy ambulances, the vice president of St. Vincent's put us up in a five-star hotel. A small group of us medics piled into an ambulance and were ferried to our luxury accommodations.

When we arrived we were greeted with curious stares from the hotel guests and staff, as we were probably the dirtiest lodgers that they had ever welcomed to their prestigious establishment. We were met by polite smiles as we entered the lobby, covered with dust and dirt. Our tired bodies and worn faces could barely manage to acknowledge what was going on around us.

It was surreal. People in fine clothes, sitting in the cocktail lounge, sipping martinis. The sounds of clinking glasses and the chatter of small talk was quite a contrast to the screams and the smashing of glass we had heard the morning before. It must have been just as surreal for the hotel guests, who were thrust into reality when the images and people they had been watching on

TV were suddenly standing before them in the flesh.

There had already been a dozen or so medics who checked into the hotel earlier. They had been sent there after serving part of the day and were about to become our replacements in the field. Most of us were given our own rooms, although several medics were doubled up.

My only thought was to take a shower, get some food, and somehow clean my clothes. I was a bit uneasy as I traveled by elevator to the thirty-second floor. I did not like heights, and I was less than overjoyed to be sleeping in a tall building the morning after September 11.

Telephone service was pretty bad, especially to New Jersey. After several attempts I finally got through to my family, only to find out that my younger daughter, Maria, had flipped herself out of the family pool and broken and dislocated four toes of her foot. She was taken to the emergency room and would have to undergo surgery later that week. Normally, I would have dropped everything and run home, but not tonight. No one was going home tonight.

I hunted around for a room service menu only to find out that both the restaurant and room service were closed and would not reopen until the morning. I was shit out of luck and becoming increasingly nauseous due to lack of sleep and lack of nourishment. Just when I was resolved to take a shower and get some rest the phone rang. It was Esteban Guerrero.

"Yo, Frankie. Can I come up for awhile and hang out?"

"I thought you were going to the bar?"

"They wouldn't let me in, bro, because I don't have a jacket and tie," he said.

"Sure. Come on up." As much as I was exhausted, I was not too eager to close my eyes.

A few minutes later there was a knock on the door and Esteban entered the room with several cans of beer.

"Today was messed up. Here." He extended his hand and offered me a drink.

"No thanks, man. I would puke."

"Be a man. I thought you were hard core."

"Really. I can't remember the last time I ate." The last thing I needed was to pour alcohol into an empty stomach churning with acid. There was an awkward silence and Esteban started to speak again.

"I love my wife."

"Of course you do."

"No I *really* love her. You know what she did?" I just looked at him blankly as I struggled to keep my eyes open.

He continued, "She gave me her vest." His wife was a Port Authority cop.

"I went down to her station and she gave me her vest. She even offered to give me her gun."

"Her gun?" My eyes popped open. I was intrigued. "What for?"

"She heard that I was rushed by patients and she was afraid I might get hurt. You know, they might trample me? So she took out her gun and offered it to me."

I just looked at him with my eyebrows raised, not knowing whether to look impressed or burst out laughing.

"That's true love. What woman would offer you her gun?" he said.

"I can think of a lot of women that would offer me a gun, but only if I promised to blow my brains out with it!" I replied.

I had this mental picture of hundreds of civilians storming the ambulance, Esteban standing on top of the rig as he opened fire into the crowd, not stopping until his magazine was empty. That would be real good for hospital public relations.

Esteban and I sat and talked for a few minutes. He was restless and was not too happy that I was not drinking with him. Again, my eyes were closing from exhaustion and the dust. He got on the phone and started calling the other rooms. Before I knew it, there were a bunch of medics in my room drinking, smoking, and using all the clean towels. My room became the party room.

Carl and I had been up at the front all day. Everybody else had gotten some R and R during the course of the day, and now they were wide awake. Sometime during the party, someone broke into the refrigerator and started drinking the beverages. In this hotel every beverage that you drank had to be paid for, and it was not cheap. A soft drink was five dollars and alcohol was ten dollars. I spied a can of peanuts and started eating them as if I had just come out of a fever. Although it was a form of food, it only made me feel more nauseous.

At about 4:30 a.m., after consuming a good five or six hundred dollars worth of booze, the party dispersed and I finally was going to get some sleep. I figured what the hell. The IRS was going to take all the money I was getting in overtime. They might as well take it out of my check, and I was happy that I treated my comrades to a good party.

I washed what I could in the bathtub and hung my clothes next to the air vent to dry. I took a long hot shower and turned on

CNN, only to see Carl and me standing with our backs to the camera in the middle of Ground Zero with fires burning all around us. It was freaky. There we were as plain as day. I wanted to call home and tell them to turn on the TV, but it seemed so insignificant. I seemed so insignificant.

I tried desperately to keep my eyes open, but it was a losing battle. I was falling asleep and praying I would not have any bad dreams. Living the tragedy was enough.

19

in the rear with the gear, 9/12

I guess the phone started ringing at about 6:30 a.m. When I finally picked up the phone it was around seven a.m. It was the secretary from the ambulance department.

"Are you alright?" the voice said.

"I'm fine. What's the matter?" thinking that there was another attack.

"We've been calling you for the past half-hour. We need to get into your room. There are other medics at the hotel and they need rooms. Why did you lock your door?"

Inadvertently, I had engaged the deadbolt after the other medics left my room.

"Security tried to get in. Boy, you're a heavy sleeper."

"Gee, I don't know why. I've only been up for about forty hours straight. A couple of hours seems like enough rest. I should be fresh as a daisy!" There was brief silence at the other end. "When do you want me to come back in?" I asked.

"Whenever you feel rested. Just unlock the door so the others can get in. We were just worried about you."

I felt bad that I had snapped at her. She probably was worried about me. I suddenly thought, what others? I had this mental picture of a platoon of medics marching into the room and waking me up again. Most medics would make noise stuffing a mattress.

I got up, took another shower, and put on my damp clothes. I was not going to get back to sleep anyway. Two and a half hours of sleep would have to do.

I walked up to Seventh Avenue and hailed a taxi. Cabs were few and far between, but I had no problem since I was in uniform. I got dropped off several blocks from the hospital because the police were not allowing civilian cars through the checkpoints.

New York had become an armed camp. There were State Police on every corner as well as police from Long Island, and even the Police Academy cadets. In the days and weeks that followed I saw police officers from as far away as Miami and Halifax, Nova Scotia.

When I arrived at the hospital the Archbishop of New York, Cardinal Egan, was holding a press conference. It had become a media circus. I was told that he had been keeping vigil at the hospital the day before and administering last rites. He had been on his way to the front on 9/11, but he had been diverted to St. Vincent's by an unnamed authority. The only clergy that I saw up at the line was a rabbi, a Protestant minister, a Catholic priest, and an Eastern Orthodox priest. Father Richard, the Eastern Orthodox priest, gave me a blessing and heard my confession at building Number Seven. They were "in the shit" just like we were, and they were comforting the sick and wounded. I just thought of my old friend Cardinal O'Connor. Sure as heck he would have been up at the front! No matter what!

Cardinal Egan is the spiritual leader of Manhattan and the New York Archdiocese. The majority of the firefighters, cops, medics and EMTs were Roman Catholic. He should have been comforting his flock on the scene.

I was not a big fan of Cardinal Egan and became less of one after his statement about the attack. When asked if the United States might have provoked the attack on 9/11 he responded by saying, "It is not necessarily that the explanation is that there have been some misdeeds on the part of the United States, but that is a possibility." This was not the time to be introspective or decide whose fault it was, especially for those of us involved in the rescues.

As I stood there in disbelief, glaring at His Eminence, two of the medic supervisors came up to me.

"We heard you had a little party in your room last night? We had to send the other guys home. They were exhausted. They looked terrible," they said.

I, of course, looked like a bouquet of roses.

"I'm not going home!" I said.

They both looked at me surprised.

"No, you're on Fifty-one X–ray with Nelson. You guys report to Chelsea Piers."

"Where is Pete?" I asked.

"Peter is riding on Five William doing 911 calls."

Nelson Rivera was a former medic student who just graduated the month before.

Nelson and I drove to the Chelsea Piers and saw a sea of ambulances from all over the country. Some of those men and women must have been driving nonstop since the Towers were hit the day before. We found an empty space among what must have been five hundred crews. This was another block party. There was free food and drink and guys joked and wandered around the area.

"So how did you do on your medic exams?" I asked Nelson.

"OK."

"Are you applying for a job at St. Vincent's?"

"No. I didn't score high enough on the state exam."

Since St. Vincent's is a teaching hospital, you have to score at least 80 percent on both parts of the state exam.

"What did you get?"

"I got a sixty-eight."

Holy shit, I thought to myself. We got a problem. He's not a paramedic.

"We gotta go back the hospital," I said.

"What's the matter?"

"Nothing. I forgot something."

When we arrived at the hospital, Nick Terranova had a puzzled look on his face.

"Back so soon?"

Nelson went inside to use the bathroom facilities, and I said, "Hey Nick, is Nelson a medic?"

"No."

"So why the hell do we have him on a medic unit?"

"What?"

"He's working an enhancement unit with me. Fifty-one X–ray."

Bill walked up to us as we were speaking.

"What's the problem?" Bill asked.

"Nelson's not a medic."

"So?"

"He's working as a medic with Frankie."

"How the hell did that happen?" Bill asked. "Hey Jim!" Bill shouted. Bill called Jim Amato, his assistant, over to the summit and they talked privately.

Jim walked over to me and said, "You and Nelson will be riding Seven King doing 911. Nelson's an EMT, right Nick?"

"Yeah, he's an EMT. All paramedic students have to be EMTs, but why the hell is he riding a St. Vinny's unit when he ain't a St. Vinny's employee, Jim?"

"We don't have enough paramedic staff and Seven King is the only BLS unit that we have. I'll pull the medics off Seven King and put them on Fifty-one X–ray."

"What do you mean we don't have the staff?"

"We sent too many people home. My mistake," Jim said. Nick shook his head.

"By the way, can you stay for a double at least?"

"I don't plan on going home until everybody's dug out," I answered. "Just get me some scrubs or something. I've been in the same clothes for three days."

"I'll work on it," Jim said.

20

back to the streets, 9/12, a.m.

I never got the hospital scrubs that Jim promised, so my first trip was to clothing stores to try to at least buy some clean skivvies.

There wasn't a store in that part of town that had plain skivvies. I wound up getting a couple of pairs of silk boxers from a store that specialized in men's lingerie. After all, it was the Village. At least it was clean, and I was probably the best-dressed medic in town in terms of my undergarments.

Our first call was for a sick patient somewhere on First Avenue. It was a street job. Since the patient turned out to be unconscious, we called for Advanced Life Support (ALS) paramedic backup after we surveyed the scene. As a basic life support unit, we carried no drugs except oxygen and epinephrine. Also arriving at the scene was a group of firemen.

The homeless man who greeted us told us that his girlfriend, who was a crack addict, fell and passed out while she was trying to urinate by a dumpster. I was less than thrilled with this call in light of 9/11, but it was a human being who was sick and maybe injured.

The firemen were less tolerant and were pissed off for getting stuck doing stupid 911 calls while their brothers were digging at the Towers. As I stood in urine and vomitus in a narrow area between the building and the dumpster, supporting the woman's neck and head, a young fireman went into a tirade.

"This is Anita. She's a neighborhood crackhead! I'm not going to stand around all day and do this bullshit!"

He did not wait around for us to give him a 55. (A 55 is a signal to fire or police department personnel that their assistance is not needed.) He just slid a backboard under her and took off for whereabouts unknown, leaving Nelson and me to try to board and collar her.

By the time we got her boarded and collared, ALS help arrived in the form of Phil Generoso and Jerry Suarez, another St. Vincent's paramedic. They heard our call for help and rushed to our aid. They had a couple of paramedic students with them, so we had no problem lifting the patient out of the narrow space and onto the ambulance.

We gave her the standard workup: IV line, dextrose, thiamine, and Narcan. As we finished pushing the Narcan, the patient was wide awake and wanted to beat us up. She became violent and had to be restrained. It took five grown men to restrain this 110-pound female.

We drove her to Beth Israel Medical Center, where the staff was disappointed that it was only a "frequent flyer" and not a victim of the Trade Center.

About one hour into the tour, Nelson told me that he had to go home. I guess doing 911 calls on a BLS ambulance was not what he had hoped his day would turn into. He wanted the high-profile ALS jobs, so we headed back to the hospital. Since

Nelson was a volunteer and not an employee of St. Vincent's, he was not required to work for any set amount of hours. It was then that I finally met up with Peter. It was a relief to see his tired face and we did the guy thing of hugging and smacking each other on the back.

"Where the hell were you?"

"Thank God you are alright. You had me worried," he answered. "They were afraid to put us together," he said.

"Yeah, we would have *really* screwed up their clusterfuck."

After Nelson went home, the supervisors put Peter and me on an ambulance together with two other medics. All of the ambulances started to resemble clown cars at the circus because of all the extra personnel.

We stopped at the garage and Peter and I went to look for my car. Just then, we saw Andrew Johns walking down the street with a medical bag slung over his shoulder.

"Hi, partner. Are you going off or coming on?" I asked.

"They're finally sending me home." Andrew replied.

"What's with the medical bag?" Peter asked.

"I'm not ready to go home yet. I'm going down to the Towers to do some search and rescue. Who knows?" he said with the tired look in his eyes of a man twice his age.

"Hey Andy. You better get some rest, brother."

"Plenty of time for that. And fishing," he added as he walked slowly and deliberately toward Ground Zero.

"He's not only a good medic, he's a good man," I said quietly. Peter nodded in agreement.

I found my car a block away without any damage. Jerry Suarez had moved my car out of the road the day before and

parked it in a safe place. Peter moved his car next to mine and
we continued to talk.

"How's your wife?" I asked.

"I thought she was going to throw herself on my car as I left.
She didn't want me to go."

"But she let you go."

"Sometimes partners are more important than wives."

21
back to the streets, 9/12, p.m.

On the afternoon of September 12 we were working 911 calls on Five William. Peter and I sat in the back with ridiculous-looking helmets on our heads while Kurt Schafer and Jack Sherwood were in the passenger's compartment looking just as silly. The helmets themselves resembled hard hats, which was not too bad. However, they had fireproof flaps that were tucked into them. When the flaps were down, they looked like a cross between the French Foreign Legion and an Easter bonnet. None of us bothered to tuck in the flaps.

The atmosphere of the city had changed in one long day. The streets were more or less deserted and the air of Lower Manhattan was hot and thick with dank smoke. Everyone was walking around with dust masks. People were doing whatever they could to help us out, whether it was moving out of the way to let our ambulances and crews pass or stopping to offer us a cold drink or food. Everyone was smiling and waving at us as we passed them by. Manhattan had a small-town atmosphere.

The first call we had was an indigent male having chest pain in the subway station on Sixth Avenue and Waverly Place, directly in front of the Duane Reade Pharmacy.

The sixty-year-old man was having shortness of breath and grabbing at his chest. We quickly secured him to a stair chair and rushed him up the subway steps.

The patient probably did not know how lucky he was to be treated by four paramedics instead of the usual two. Peter and I had to step back because there was not enough room in the ambulance for four medics or four egos. We watched as the senior medics blew an IV line and fiddled with the monitor. Later, I wound up getting the IV line. Peter had the nitro and aspirin already out. Jack Sherwood was impressed that we had our act together and looked proudly at his former students as we treated the patient. Jack was one of the preceptors when Peter and I were in medic school. He stepped back and let us finish the call, but Kurt Schafer, the other senior medic, looked pissed off that we were handling things competently.

"You know, there isn't enough room in the back of the ambulance for the four of us," he said.

"Then maybe we should get in the front and let the rookies handle this call," Jack said.

To Jack, anyone who did not have as much experience as he did was a rookie. I don't think he was pulling rank with us as much as he was giving Schafer a dignified way to "save face" without bruising his ego.

In reality, it is no big deal when you miss an IV line. Sometimes the catheter kinks, sometimes you hit a valve in a vein, and sometimes a patient has weak veins. Sometimes you just miss.

That is why you have a partner. On the days when you cannot get a line, 99.99 percent of the time your partner can. Somehow, it always works that way. If you both cannot get the line, chances are it cannot be gotten. The worst case is that a central line will have to be inserted at the hospital. If you absolutely need to get a line in, in a cardiac arrest, for example, there are always the external jugular veins or the feet.

Kurt, like most medics, doesn't like to miss an IV line. His temper flared some more when Peter not only diagnosed that the patient was having a heart attack but pinpointed the area of the heart that was being damaged.

"He is having an inferior wall MI and has anterior-septal wall ischemia," said Peter.

Jack laughed and said, "Thank you, Doctor Castellano."

Kurt, now having his ego totally bashed, said, "We don't need to know that. All we need to know is that he has chest pain and he is infarcting."

22

another block party, 9/12

Upon our arrival at the hospital, we were met with another wave of health care workers still desperately waiting for survivors from the crash. We saw the frustration and disappointment on their faces when they saw us take our homeless patient out of the ambulance. It would be a scene that would be repeated time after time in the next few days.

After writing up the paperwork, we headed back in the ambulance, winding our way down toward Ground Zero. This time we did not get too far. We made our way down Varick Street to North Moore Street, where the Salvation Army courtesy stands were now set up along the sidewalks, resembling a street fair.

Even McDonald's had a booth, generously giving away free food. There was a huge roadblock and checkpoint at the intersection of Varick and North Moore Streets. No vehicles were able to pass. Even if cars did gain access, the street was crowded with emergency workers on foot, which made it virtually impassable.

Everyone was wearing some sort of protective mask, so faces were indistinguishable. The streets were wet with water from being constantly hosed down to alleviate the flying dust. It was a muddy, dank mess and the smell was like a moldy urban cellar.

Our crew of four stepped out of the vehicle and walked up to another St. Vincent's ambulance crew that was parked on the other side of the street. They were just standing there, waiting for the chance to go down to where the Towers once stood.

I took off my protective mask and lit up a cigarette. One of the other crew members started to admonish me in a high-pitched voice. "I can't believe that in the middle of all this you are still smoking," she shouted through her mask.

"After everything that happened, I'm lucky that I'm not on a crack pipe," I shouted back.

I could not recognize who it was because of the protective facegear, but after noticing protruding long strawberry-blonde locks I realized it was Regina Ryan.

Regina is a full–time nurse in Connecticut. She occasionally works at St. Vincent's and was one of the only per diem medics to help out during the crisis. A per diem medic usually works only one tour a week and holds a full-time position someplace else.

Regina also teaches part-time in the paramedic school at St. Vincent's. She is a beautiful woman and once had been asked to pose for *Playboy* magazine, when she was in college. As a good Catholic and the daughter of a retired firefighter, she flatly refused.

I always enjoyed riding in the ambulance with Regina when I was a student because, being a teacher, she let me practice clinical skills with patients.

I got into a little difficulty at medic school when a rumor reached the administration that Regina and I were having an affair. I remember the program director of the school, Nick Terranova, calling me into the office and explaining to me that St. Vincent's was a Catholic hospital and I should not be sleeping with an instructor. Nick and another hospital administrator warned me that I could be expelled for my alleged behavior.

Regina really felt the burden of it, although I think things really got blown way out of proportion. For her sake, I did not ride with her anymore as a student.

She hugged me, and Peter said, "I knew something was going on with you two."

I knew that Peter was just teasing, but I doubt that Regina did. She took everything literally. She gave him a love tap.

"Don't hit him, he likes it," I said. She then hit me.

"More, more," I said.

Our crew walked back to the ambulance and we spent the rest of the tour trying to do something useful. We looked everywhere for patients to treat, even ones with minor cuts and scrapes. We handed out dust masks to anyone we saw with an exposed face.

Everywhere we went civilians were feeding us and giving us free refreshments. They moved out of our way as we drove down the street. They smiled and waved and even applauded.

The people in Chelsea, Tribeca, and Greenwich Village were especially great. The locals set up a stand right on Eleventh Street next to the hospital. They manned it twenty-four hours a day. They had coffee that Starbuck's donated and food from local restaurants and stores. There was so much food donated to the hospital that we had to get cars to take it away and send it to the

112

needy of the city or down to the workers at the Pile.

Actors and celebrities who lived in New York came to the hospital to volunteer their services. I personally saw Sigourney Weaver and Kathleen Turner doing manual labor. I am told that dozens more people from the entertainment community helped out.

Kim Raver, an actress who plays a paramedic on the television show *Third Watch,* was down at the hospital performing menial tasks and boosting morale. She helped wash the dirty boots of emergency workers and brought us bottles of water as we sat outside of the hospital. Sometimes she would just sit and hold hands and talk to us. Kim was volunteering from the very beginning of the crisis. It was not a photo op for those people. They were just ordinary New Yorkers helping out in an extraordinary way.

In the early days after 9/11 there was a line a block long with people volunteering to give blood. I never saw New Yorkers so united or behave so kindly to one another.

23

fifteen minutes, 9/12

Zero Five William?" The radio squawked.

"Five Willie," they answered.

"Five William, where is your current location?" Dispatch asked.

"Fourteen and Nine, Central," they replied.

"Then why is your vehicle seventeen-seventy-eight parked on West Street?"

"That is not our vehicle, Central. It has been parked there since Tuesday morning."

For the last two days the crews of Five William had been getting calls for vehicle 1778—the ambulance that Ned and Andrew used on the eleventh—and it was still at Ground Zero. Because vehicle 1778 had never logged off, Central Dispatch still had ambulance 1778 assigned to unit Five William. Dispatch was concerned about the whereabouts of the crew. No matter how many times Central Dispatch was told the crew was alright and in a different bus, a new dispatcher would log on or a new conditions boss would pass by vehicle 1778 and would call Five William for an update. It became a running gag, and this went on almost every hour on the hour.

My fifteen minutes of fame came early in the evening of September 12. I was partnered with Regina Ryan on Five

William. We were checking out the ambulance before we went into service as night was falling. Sean Anderson, who was in charge of publicity for the hospital, stepped up to the ambulance. He asked me if I would do some interviews. "It would be really good for the hospital," he added.

"Thanks for thinking about me, Sean, but I'm going into service soon."

I would rather have eaten glass than do an interview. I do not know if Sean asked me to be interviewed because of my acting background or because I was the only medic who would be dumb enough to stand in front of a camera. I am not good at that sort of thing. When I act I have the anonymity of the stage, with costumes, lights, makeup, and a script. I am someone else. In an interview you are using your own words. You are you. Remembering my show business days, I would either wind up sticking my foot in my mouth or looking like a pompous ass.

Sean was disappointed, but he was persistent. He returned in a few minutes with another man in a suit.

"I am Dr. Goldwyn," the handsome middle-aged man said.

"Frank Rella," I said, extending my hand.

"Senior vice president of the hospital," Sean added.

"Listen Frank, we would appreciate it if you would do an interview for the hospital," Goldwyn requested politely.

Realizing that Dr. Goldwyn was pretty much in charge of the hospital, it would not be a good idea to say no.

"Let me just square it with my supervisor, sir," I said to Dr. Goldwyn.

I figured that I would let the on-duty supervisor say no, so I went into Gabe Abram's office.

"Look, there are a couple of suits from the hospital outside and they want me to do an interview," I told Gabe. I left out the fact that Goldwyn was one of the people who asked me. I figured that Gabe would tell me that I could not do the interview and that would be that.

"That sounds OK, but stay available in case you get called," he said.

I told Regina that I was going to do the interview and I assumed that she understood that we were not going into service for a while, since we still had some time before our shift began.

In the middle of the interview with *Good Morning America,* Regina came into full view of the television camera and started screaming.

"They're calling for us!"

I stopped talking into the camera. "Who's calling for us? We're not in service yet!"

"Dispatch. They are calling for Five William and nobody is answering. They want to know what vehicle we're in. They probably have a job waiting."

I knew that it was our hourly bullshit call about vehicle 1778. Regina would not shut up about it as much as I tried to explain it to her. Luckily the interview was being taped or we would have looked like complete jackasses. Finally, I excused myself and walked back to the ambulance to explain the situation to Central on the radio.

Just as I finished the interview, a reporter from Reuters started pounding me with questions. He was trying to get me to state that there were patients being found in the rubble. He wanted me to commit to a number and asked, "Can you say exactly how many people were found?" He asked the same question in many different ways.

Finally, I said, "I've heard lots of rumors, but I don't know if any of them are true. I'm not going to give you a number just so you can write it on your note pad. I wouldn't want to give any false hopes to the families of the victims or to the public."

Since he was not getting what he wanted, the interview was terminated. Now I was ready to go into service. But wait! Dan Rather wanted to interview me on live TV.

I looked squarely at Gabe Abrams and took him aside. "I have fifteen minutes before the tour officially starts and I swear to Christ I'm walking off camera at that precise moment!"

He looked at me in disbelief while sweat was pouring down his forehead. The last thing he wanted to do was to make an enemy with the senior vice president of the hospital. I had Gabe call and tell Central Dispatch that Five William, tour three, would be going into service on time.

A production assistant wired me for sound and stood there waiting for Dan Rather to speak. Suddenly I heard someone say, "Fifteen seconds to interview," then "ten seconds to interview," then "five, four, three, two, one."

By this time I had practically no voice left. The dust from Ground Zero had given me a case of acute laryngitis, so I was growling into the microphone to answer Dan Rather's questions.

"With us now is one of the thousands of brave people risking their lives in the rescue effort, Frank Rella. Mr. Rella is a paramedic," he began. "Thank you for joining us. Our admiration for what you are doing knows no bounds."

I thought to myself, wow! That's Dan Rather at the other end of this hookup. What the hell am I doing here and why is he thanking me? Somebody else should be doing this interview with him.

He continued to question me. "How eerie is it to be working under these circumstances?"

I swallowed to try to clear my throat, but it sounded as if I gargled with Drano. "Well, sir, it's nothing that you can ever train for or you can ever anticipate. It's part of our lives. I mean, we come here [to the city] every day and try to do the best we can for people, but this is nothing that you can ever anticipate happening."

"What's the worst of it?" Rather asked.

"The worst of it is not being able to find patients or our brothers, the firefighters or the police who have been lost. I mean, we're here to save people. And especially paramedics and EMTs, we're here to treat patients and we can't find any patients," I answered, finding myself getting emotional while I was talking. Doing everything to hold in my feelings.

Rather asked, "How realistic is it to believe that at this late time, there may still be people alive in the debris, Mr. Rella?"

"Well sir, I think it is the only thing that really can keep us going. Just saying that there are people there (under the debris) and we're going to get them out and we're going to make sure that we'll stay here until it's done."

"You do or do not have a sense of real and present danger as you go about this work?" Rather queried.

"Well, I don't think any of us think about that. I think somebody being trapped is more important than us being afraid. I mean, anybody who doesn't fear is crazy, but we don't let that fear get to us. The people that were out there (at Ground Zero) and are still out there are going to go back in there and, at risk of their own personal safety, they'll do what they have to do. They'll do their jobs and they'll do them well."

"You say they'll do their jobs and do them well? You'll do your job and you'll do it well, Mr. Rella."

He then signed off, "Frank Rella—paramedic. One of our heroes. Thank you."

I am told that he then had to hold back tears as he spoke his last words, "You're watching continuing CBS News coverage of the attack on America."

Within minutes, several phone calls came in to the public relations office of St. Vincent's. Dan Rather had been genuinely touched by what I said and CBS called to thank the hospital. "Who was the young man who made Dan Rather cry?" the director of CBS Evening News asked.

The next call was from Peter Jennings' office at ABC. He wanted to do an interview with me at their studios the next morning.

Another was from Oprah Winfrey's office, asking to do an interview with me.

"How about that, Frank?" said Sean Anderson. "This is more than your fifteen minutes of fame! Just think of the good you will be doing for the hospital, and it is your big chance. I told them that you are an actor and a singer. Think what this could mean for your career. We can get lots of public appearances lined up for you."

"Sean, at any other time I would jump at something like this, but this is not what this is all about. I don't want to capitalize on all this misery. Besides, what the hell did I do?"

"It's not what you did, it's what you represent," he answered.

"The city needs heroes. You look like a hero and damn it, you did more than you know!"

"All the heroes are under the rubble at Ground Zero. The rest of us were just doing our jobs!"

Sean looked at me, speechless.

"Yesterday morning, I stopped being an actor and started being a paramedic. I'm going to stay a paramedic, at least for the duration," I said.

At that moment, Sean and I became real friends.

"You're OK, Frank."

He shook my hand tightly and smiled.

"You're OK too, Sean."

Suddenly Sean stopped being a PR guy. We were two people who were just trying to do the right thing. I admit that I probably would have gotten a lot of press, and it could have skyrocketed my performing career. But right then the only thing that was important to me was riding in my ambulance and finding patients to help.

Finally, Regina and I went into service. The only call we got was from an AIDS center late in the shift. The call was for a middle-aged woman who had a fever. There was nothing much for us to do other than transport her to the hospital.

As the tour came to a close, I realized that I had been working for sixteen hours. I was wondering if they were going to send me to the hotel again. I really did not want to go off duty yet. Regina was going to do the overnight shift, so I volunteered to stay and work another eight hours with her. I enjoyed working with her because she would never bitch about getting any ambulance call. No matter what type of call we got, she was always happy to help another human being. Besides, I did not want to be at the hotel, sleeping, when they finally started pulling patients out of the ruins.

24
night shift, 9/13

Regina and I went back to the ambulance office to get fresh batteries for our radios and something to eat.

When I opened the office door, Carl was sitting with Gabe Abrams and they looked like they were up to something. Carl had gone home early that morning. He was wide awake and looking well rested. By the time I was starting the overnight shift on Thursday morning, I had already been in New York City for the better part of three and a half days.

Carl arranged with Gabe to replace Regina and work with me. After being on the ambulance for sixteen hours that day, the last thing I wanted to do was to drive around all night and tech. Carl was in full "commander mode," which meant he would be driving, talking on the radio, talking on the Nextel, playing with the onboard computer, and being a resident expert. I was in no mood. Regina was disappointed that she was being sent home and so was I.

The night went pretty much as I expected. We wandered around all of Lower Manhattan, first to the garage, then as close to Ground Zero as we could get, and finally back to the hospital. We were assigned to the normal eighty–nine of Three Victor,

Sixth Avenue and West Fourth Street, but there were no conditions bosses to check up on us. All of the EMS officers were either at the central command post or in or around Ground Zero. If a call came in we could get anywhere in Lower Manhattan in a matter of minutes, because there were hardly any civilian cars on the streets. Everything was blocked off from the Chelsea Piers on West Twenty-third Street to the Battery Tunnel at the southernmost tip of Manhattan. Lower Manhattan was a ghost town.

Carl and I listened attentively to the radio and visited every block party that we passed. At every big intersection there were people gathered, holding vigil and with food and drink in hand, anxious to give their supplies away to any emergency vehicle that passed. We were America's guests. All I wanted to do was find a quiet spot where I could rest my eyes and monitor the radio until the shift ended.

The only call of the night came at the end of our shift. It was in Alphabet City, in the projects.

When we arrived in the apartment of our patient, a woman in her forties was complaining of difficulty breathing.

"All the dust from Ground Zero gathered in my apartment. It made me sick."

Her lungs sounded clear, but we put her on oxygen and transported her to Bellevue.

By the time we got back for the tour change, it was after nine a.m. I volunteered for another tour, but the supervisors ordered me off duty.

As I drove up to the entrance of the Holland Tunnel, on my way home, I was stopped by a young police officer. The precinct number on his collar indicated that he was from outside of Manhattan. I showed him my badge and ID card.

"Sorry, you can't go through the tunnel. Emergency personnel only."

"I'm a city paramedic from St. Vincent's," I said.

"Sorry. We aren't even letting sanitation workers through. Only emergency workers!"

"Do me a favor. Call the Sixth or First Precinct and tell them that you have a Vinny's medic sitting at the tunnel waiting to go through."

Just then, another young police officer walked over. He was from the Sixth Precinct. It was Richie DiNardio. "Where are you going? Leaving so soon?" he asked.

"I'm trying to. Thank God you're OK."

"Geeze, you look like shit! You better get some sleep." He turned to the other officer and said, "Any medics coming through can use the tunnel."

The long night's journey into day was finally coming to an end. I was finishing the trip home that began on the morning of September 11. I had the radio tuned to News Radio eight–eighty. I was trying to find out what happened in the past two days. Were we at war? How many people did they say made it out of the Towers? Was anyone found yet in the rubble?

Along the New Jersey Turnpike the State Police were out in full force. There were roadblocks and lines of emergency vehicles heading into the city.

The problems that clouded my head on my drive home on the morning of 9/11 were now the furthest things from my mind. They seemed inconsequential in light of what had happened.

All I wanted to do was hug my daughters and tell them that I was alright. I wanted to shower and rest up for the work that was ahead of me.

I stopped at the local coffee shop on the way to my house. The people on line all stepped aside and offered me their place and muttered words of thanks. The young man at the counter refused to take my money as he handed me a large cup of coffee.

As I turned the corner to my house I saw a large American flag draped on the side of it. Tears started to swell up in my eyes. I took a couple of deep breaths.

My neighbor, a New Jersey police officer, was mowing my lawn. He turned off the engine when he saw my Jeep.

"I didn't know when you would be back. I just wanted to do something to help out."

25

home front, 9/13–9/14

I arrived home in Old Bridge just in time to see my daughter Maria off to her surgery. Both of my daughters hugged me tightly as I got out of the car.

Maria was undergoing general anesthesia for repositioning the bones in her foot. Luckily, when they reset her bones, pins were not needed and she eventually regained full use of her foot.

My mother made me something to eat and I tried to get some sleep. In the first few months after the crash I could not sleep more than an hour at a time. I would wake up with the least little sound. I should have realized that I needed some counseling, or at the very least, the critical stress debriefing the hospital later gave, but I was not the type to talk about my problems with others and tried to brush them off.

I spent most of the day tossing and turning. I watched television a lot, trying to grasp the enormity of the events, and monitored my police scanner to see if anything serious was happening in Manhattan. My mother and I watched the religious service that was attended by the president and his family. I was moved, not so much by the religious aspect, but by the care and kindness of our president.

Although exhausted mentally and physically, all I wanted to do was get back into the city. To keep my mind off it, I washed all of the crud off of my car and packed a bag with clean uniforms and underwear. If I was going to get stuck in the city again, I was going to have enough clean clothes for the duration.

I went to a local uniform shop and bought a "buff" light for my car. I was not going to drive to the next mass casualty incident with my hand sticking out of the window. I also installed a two-way radio.

Unbeknown to me, I started to exhibit signs of stress reaction, or, to give it a fancy name, posttraumatic stress disorder. Looking back, I could see that I was fatigued, anxious, angry, had a poor attention span and heightened alertness. I was blaming Tammy for my daughter's accident. I was obsessed with trying to turn my car into a tactical vehicle. I had nightmares and intrusive images.

The most disturbing thing, aside from grief, was the tremendous sense of guilt that I felt. First of all, for not being able to do more and, second, for being alive while so many others had died.

I also began lashing out at others, not in a violent way, but I did not want to hear about the little problems that people were going through in their everyday lives. I also did not want to spend time with anyone. I was comforted by the fact that I had at least two friends, Tara and Todd, who took the time out to call me, but it would be weeks before I would call them and thank them. All I wanted to do was sit in my ambulance and wait for the big call.

The media was making heroic icons of the NYPD and

FDNY, deservedly, since they had the most losses apart from civilians. But the tragedy was not just about them or other uniformed services. It was about secretaries and office workers, mothers and fathers.

The less publicized funerals of 9/11 were in communities all over the country. In my hometown, weeks later, we buried not fewer than five victims of the terrorist attack.

It is true that the uniformed workers who lost their lives did it in the service of others. While people were running out of the buildings, uniformed service workers were running in! However, how many families were torn apart? How many orphans were produced? And what about the living? What about the law enforcement officers, firefighters, and emergency medical personnel that have to carry on and take with them the memory of their brothers and sisters that they could not get to and could not help? How many relationships were ended because one partner became mentally and physically distant and could not deal with the present moment? How long can a person love you if they are getting nothing in return for weeks and months? Can you push those you love away indefinitely before they push you away out of frustration or self-preservation?

Although I believe firmly that life on earth is a passage that eventually leads to the Kingdom of Heaven, the loss of life is filled with sadness for the living. Even though I believe that I will see my infant son, my younger brother, grandparents, and great-grandparents, the event of their deaths was devastating and a source of major sadness in my life. The only difference was that their deaths were expected. Nothing could be compared to the unexpected death of a loved one.

I was forever changed on that hot summer day in September. In a way I think I lost whatever innocence I had left. And in another way I think I became more innocent, more loving, and more caring.

The ONLY good thing that might have come out of this catastrophe is the way we treat each other; how we love each other and appreciate who each person is and what they do. Now people look at firefighters and respect the lives that they lead. They look at police officers and realize that there is a name and face connected to a uniform. They look at the medics and EMTs in the ambulance and realize that when the lights are flashing and the sirens are sounding, they are on their way, eager to help save someone's life.

26

manhole covers in the sky, 9/14

I loaded up my car and headed toward the city. It was Friday night of the first week of the attack.

Earlier that day I went to the recruiting office of the New Jersey Army National Guard and filled out my enlistment papers. If there was going to be a war, I did not want to be left out of the action. I was already forty-two years old, but with my prior military service I was still eligible to serve. The only thing that might have been an impediment was the heart attack I suffered four years before.

Meanwhile, I would serve the 911 system of the City of New York. It was too early to lose hope for survivors. People in similar situations were known to survive for weeks.

There was little activity on the New Jersey Turnpike this time. The clerk at the toll booth, seeing that I was in uniform, gave me a special toll pass. "You're an emergency worker. You don't pay."

From Jersey City, I looked at the skyline of New York. In the middle of the landscape there were bright lights with heavy smoke pouring out of the ground. The surrounding buildings were dark and resembled gravestones. Ground Zero was truly a cemetery.

Near the Holland Tunnel there was a roadblock manned by State Police. As I approached I put on my blue emergency light to give the troopers the heads up. They looked at my credentials and let me pass. "Have a safe night, brother."

Once again I was a lone vehicle heading towards a crippled city.

It was less eerie than my previous solo trip through the Lincoln Tunnel, but I was queasy when I thought of what had happened to my beautiful city and the souls that might be lying under the pile, hopefully still alive.

The ambulance garage was closed. All crews would be turning out of the hospital, so we were allowed to park our cars anywhere we wished. No one would be giving us tickets with an EMS ID in our windows. The block party was continuing in full force and there were still plenty of television crews assembled across Seventh Avenue.

I parked my Jeep on Greenwich Avenue and saw Peter and Carl checking out their ambulance. Both looked disgruntled and war weary.

"This is nonsense," Peter groused.

"They have us doing 911 calls while FDNY-EMS and out-of-town vollies are stationed down at Ground Zero," Carl added.

Gracie was checking out our bus while I was talking to the boys.

Graciela "Gracie" Flores was the shortest medic in the garage, but she was like Atom Ant in the cartoons. She could carry ten times her weight. At times, working with Gracie was like watching a performance of a one-man band.

Simultaneously, she would start an IV line and draw up drugs into syringes. With her one hand she would stop a bleeding artery and take a blood pressure, while the other hand was writing up the paperwork. She would carry the cardiac monitor with one arm and the oxygen bag with the other, while pulling the stretcher with her feet. Out of generosity, Gracie insisted on doing it all.

Her earliest experiences as a paramedic were with the private ambulance service. She was accustomed to being a solo medic with an EMT driver. She would sometimes forget that she was now partnered up with another medic, and so had a tough time sharing responsibilities. None of this was out of malice. She didn't have a mean bone in her body; it was just a habit that she had a hard time shaking.

Gracie is a kind soul and a hard worker. A South American immigrant and divorced woman with a young child, she struggled to learn the English language and study for a good-paying job. In addition to becoming a paramedic, she holds two degrees and is a certified teacher. All of the medics on the overnight shift are very protective of her, although she can more than hold her own with her male counterparts.

Later on in the evening, Gracie and I bypassed a couple of checkpoints and ended up near Ground Zero. The streets were pretty much deserted and we could make it anywhere in our area within minutes. Besides, there were still no conditions bosses around to really check up on us. Carl and Peter met up with us. We were sitting somewhere on West Broadway when we heard an explosion.

Holy shit! We're getting hit again! we all thought. Before we could realize what was happening there was another explosion. This time we saw what the source was. Manhole covers were flying into the air and flames were shooting out from underground New York. Shortly before the explosions, we had passed a bunch of Con Ed workers and when we looked back they were gone.

Quickly I got on the radio and called it in.

"Zero Five William for the priority."

The dispatcher asked, "What is your current situation Five William?"

"Five William. In the vicinity of West Bee-way and Chambers. Explosions. Possible devices."

"Five William. Proceed with caution. Check and advise."

"Five William, Ten-four," I answered.

We parked our vehicles a block away and I got out of my vehicle and started to walk towards one of the holes.

"Gracie. Stay in the ambulance," I ordered. I told Gracie to stay in the vehicle in case something happened to me. I really wanted her to stay someplace safe. There was no reason for both of us to buy the farm, and she was a single parent.

Carl stuck his head out of the other ambulance and started talking to me. "Call for ESU. Didn't you learn anything from nine-eleven?" he lectured.

"Hey Carl. You're not my supervisor. If you don't want to come with me, stay in the rear with the gear!" I shouted, feeling somewhat sorry that I snapped at him.

As I walked away from the vehicle toward the fiery holes in the ground, Peter followed me.

"Pete, keep back. I don't want to make your wife a widow."

"Screw you. I'm coming with you!"

"Seriously, if the shit hits the fan you're the only one I want to drag my ass out! I'll be careful," I replied.

"Pete don't be stupid. Don't let Frankie go," Carl called out.

"You should know by this time that no one can stop that marine! Pull the bus back and wait for me," Peter ordered Carl.

"Stay behind, Peter," I warned as I continued walking towards the holes.

"I'm just a few steps behind you, partner," Peter said.

Peter kept a half a block behind me. I wished he was back in the ambulance with Carl, but Peter has a hard head, too.

As I trotted down the street, other manhole covers started exploding. It was not a safe place to be. I went to the first hole and shone my flashlight into the darkness, but there was nothing but smoke and stinky sewer gas. I saw a Con Ed worker in the distance.

"Are there any workers in the hole?" I asked.

"I don't know," he replied.

I went to the next hole and then to the next, and then to the next. Each time I shone my light I was looking into nothingness. One of the holes had an active fire that singed the brim of my baseball cap.

Just as I was about to go down into the final hole where we first saw the workers, a Con Ed truck pulled up next to me.

"Hey, buddy. There are no workers down there. We heard your call over the radio. Everybody's accounted for."

A Con Ed worker later explained that underground buildup of sewer gas unrelated to 9/11 caused the explosions.

27

murray street triage

In the next days, while there was still hope for survivors, we would sneak down to Ground Zero every night.

I had been working one evening with Becky Stavros. I was on the first leg of a double shift that would take me into a tour one, midnight-to-eight, shift. Becky was not your ordinary medic. She was not your ordinary person. She was kind of an EDP, in large part due to her shopping addiction. She would risk putting herself out of service to go to Bed, Bath and Beyond. I have no idea how she could possibly fit all the stuff she bought into her two-bedroom town house, but somehow she managed. I imagined her house cluttered with tchatchkes and she and her husband sleeping on top of a pile.

She also had the photography habit. She was always snapping pictures, running to the pharmacy for the prints and showing them to you.

In order to get to Ground Zero, Becky would drive along and pick up workers heading down to the Pile. When she was stopped she would just tell the police officers that she was taking workers to the front, and they would let her through. Actually, security was pretty lax in the first couple of weeks. Most of the checkpoints were manned by NYPD from the area and they knew who we were. The police would still routinely check the back of our ambulances, but they would not hassle us about going up to the front.

We drove down to Greenwich and Murray Streets and were right smack in view of the ruins of building Number Seven. It was the first time I had seen the building that almost took my life, minus the dust and smoke. In front of the building were several fire trucks and ladders pouring water onto the residual flames. It was a fire company from Toronto, Canada. Our friends from up north were freeing up their indigenous firefighter brothers so the latter could dig in the Pile.

An FDNY battalion chief who looked like he was about one hundred years old was standing directly in front of the crash site. He looked up and smiled. I thought we were going to get a tongue lashing for being somewhere that we were not supposed to be. I was also reluctant to go up to the front because of Becky's intent to take pictures. I doubt if anybody would have been too friendly if she was snapping pictures while the rescue workers were trying to do their jobs. When the camera flashed, I looked at the old chief and said, "Sorry."

He said, "Why? You earned it." He looked at Becky's patch. "St. Vinny's medics. This is your building."

We walked back toward Chambers Street and I saw a group of chairs and a couple of desks that some emergency workers must have set up for themselves to rest on. It was refuse from the office buildings that had collapsed. I wondered what man or woman once sat at those desks and in those chairs. Were they alive or dead? Were they still under the rubble, and when were we going to get them out?

Written on a piece of cardboard was a sign that said:
Building 7 Cafe
MENU
Breakfast-Water
Lunch-Water
Dinner-Water
Snack-Water

Was humor coming back into the world? I am sure that the author of the sign meant no disrespect, and after all, it was building Number Seven. Nobody died in building Number Seven. If it had been the other two Towers I doubt if there would have been such levity. Was it alright to smile again? I did not feel like I wanted to. I felt like I just got the shit kicked out of me.

Becky and I walked across Murray Street and on to West Street. I was absolutely insistent that she did not take any pictures at the two main Towers. "What, are you a coward? Are you scared to go up there?" she said.

"I just don't want your sorry body to get arrested."

As we got a block away from the Pile, an overweight EMS lieutenant approached us. "What are you doing up here?" he asked. He looked as if he had just arrived at the front, with his starched shirt and newly issued jacket. He had a patch from a station in Canarsie, Brooklyn. He also was wearing the patch of an EMT.

"We're paramedics from St. Vincent's," I replied. He looked at me, confused. "This is our area, Lieutenant," I said.

"Not any more. We've been assigned here. We don't need any sightseers at the front."

Ignoring him, Becky and I continued to walk toward the Towers. Becky was oblivious to the encounter as she busily snapped pictures and waved at the workers passing us by. She was like a kid at Disneyland and the workers were more than happy to have a pretty girl smile at them.

Luckily, Becky ran out of film before we actually made it to the Towers. While passing the pudgy lieutenant on our way back to the ambulance, I heard him talking on a cell phone, sounding like he was reporting us to the Manhattan switchboard.

We turned the corner on Greenwich and saw a group of EMTs and an EMS lieutenant in a small store. We went in and asked the lieutenant what was going on.

"This is the Murray Street Triage. If anything happens, we're right here."

Here was a bunch of worn-out EMTs waiting desperately to do something. It was dirty and dank and the whole atmosphere was depressing. No one was talking, just whispering. It looked like an old-time saloon in the Wild West, except there was no booze.

"Do you want me to have you assigned here? Just park your vehicle next to the MERV," said the incredibly tired-looking lieutenant.

"No thanks. We're just visiting. We're doing 911."

He didn't even look up. He just nodded as we were leaving.

It was at that point that my heart really sank and I started losing hope. A group of sad people in a world turned upside down. God have mercy on us all!

28
back to ground zero

A few weeks after the crash, BEMS requested that St. Vincent's supply a unit to Ground Zero on a regular basis. Designated Sixty Victor, it would be a twelve-hour shift and would sit right on Liberty Street overlooking the Pile. FDNY-EMS did not have the personnel to staff the rescue operation alone, and they came pleading to the voluntary hospitals for help.

My first tour on Sixty Victor was with Jack Sherwood. We sat on Liberty Street and watched the armies of men filing in and out of the Pile, hoping to recover something or someone. We were the only paramedic unit there along with the assigned EMT units, which were mostly out-of-town volunteer first-aid companies.

Whenever there was an injury, the Ground Zero unit would take the patient up to Bellevue, and another EMT enhancement unit that was deployed at the Chelsea Piers would replace it at the Pile. The Chelsea Piers was beginning to thin out. Volunteers had to go back home and get on with their lives and their real jobs.

Morale was probably at rock bottom. Everyone was frustrated that there was nothing to do, and the reality set in that there were going to be few patients to treat. Tedium turned into apathy; monotony turned into boredom.

In the harbor nearby sat the *Spirit of New York*, a large yacht that was used for day trips. It had been voluntarily pressed into service at the beginning of the crisis and provided hot meals to the workers, as well as had shower facilities and even a resident massage therapist.

Every uniformed service was represented in the dining area: FDNY, NYPD, ESU, Corrections ESU, Court Officers, State Police, Postal Police, Port Authority, firefighters, EMS, and various federal agencies.

The courtyard of the surrounding buildings resembled a large flea market. There were tables set up for blocks on end giving away free gear, food, clothing, footwear, and sundries, all items donated by the good people of America. Becky was in her glory. Free shopping! Bed, Bath and Beyond stock plummeted during those weeks.

The variety-store atmosphere was occasionally interrupted when small utility vehicles would pass with a stretcher and a full body bag. Sadly, even this became a normal part of the routine. Ground Zero was now a factory of excavation and corpse processing.

The expressions on people's faces changed over the first few weeks. It went from shock to disbelief, and from resolve to acceptance. Nothing was left to do but wait. Wait and see what we would dig up.

I walked to the checkpoint leading to the work area overlooking West Street. Two young marines stood there guarding the entrance. I saw Peter and myself twenty years ago. I imagined what we would think as young men and what we would feel. It was too long ago, but I could see both of us in their young bodies and stern faces, standing tall. Proud of the honor of guarding such a sacred site.

I walked up to them. "You want a cigarette, marine?" I asked the sergeant. "Sorry sir, I don't smoke," he said.

"Don't call me sir. I work for a living," I said. This was the standard Marine Corps enlisted man's answer when he was called sir. "How about you, Corporal?"

"No thanks, sir. I don't smoke, either."

"Former marine?" asked the sergeant. I nodded. "*Semper fi,*" he added. (*Semper Fi* is short for *Semper Fidelis,* the Marine Corps motto.)

"*Semper Fi,*" I replied. "What's the Marine Corps coming to? NCOs who don't smoke?"

"That's the old Marine Corps. We're trying to phase old guys like that out."

Old guys? I thought. Things had really changed. As I puffed on my cigarette and studied the Pile, I wondered if they had changed for the better.

29
critical stress debriefing

Jack Sherwood and I made our way back to the hospital after spending the night at the Pile. We were pretty tired after twelve hours of doing nothing but walking around, smoking cigarettes, and eating spicy Salvation Army food. The last thing I wanted to do was attend a critical stress debriefing, though I realize now that I was in denial. I pictured everyone in the ambulance department sitting in a circle, holding hands and singing "Kumbaya."

St. Vincent's Hospital called in some counselors from another hospital to talk to us about our feelings and help us make some sense of what had happened. As I said before, I am not really good about talking about my problems one-on-one, let alone in a room full of people. I just wanted to go home and go to bed. I was beat.

When we got to the hospital, Bill Batista approached me, looking as if he was going to ask me to stay for another twelve hours. "Frank. Would you mind going back to Ground Zero and taking some equipment to the Sixty Victor crew? The crew left the hospital without their hand-held radios."

"What ambulance should I take?" I asked without hesitation.

"Take the command car."

Because I wanted to skip out of the group therapy session, I jumped at the chance of having a legitimate excuse. It was also another opportunity to go back down to the Pile in the hope that they would find someone alive while I was down there. Besides, they were letting me take the command car, which was a really cool SUV.

I had no trouble getting up to the front in the command car. Thinking that I was an EMS officer, they passed me through checkpoint after checkpoint. The only thing that was missing was the salutes. I stopped briefly at North Moore Street where a lady was kind enough to give me a bag of McDonald's food. I thought the crew would appreciate eating "real" junk food while having to sit in one spot for twelve hours.

When I arrived at the front, I parked on Liberty Street. I was really on a high until a sanitation worker approached me.

"Hey. Move your damn car out of the way!" he ordered.

Obviously he did not understand the importance of my position. I gave the crew the radios and the food and got out of the way so the garbage man would not run me over.

When I got back to the hospital, the critical stress debriefing was still in session. Damn, I thought to myself. I almost got out of it.

In the hospital conference room, a sea of faces stared at me.

"Do you want to talk about something, Frank?" Bill asked in the quiet voice of a concerned parent.

"Why, did I do something wrong?" I have a bad habit of trying to joke around when others are trying to be serious, sort of like making someone laugh in church.

A strange woman asked, "Is anything bothering you?"

I looked at her for a moment. "A lot is bothering me."

"Why don't you tell us?"

"Well, I need a shower and a decent meal and about a month off from work."

Bill was holding in a laugh and Gabe was shocked at my response.

"No. I mean is anything bothering you about what happened on the eleventh?"

"We were told that you were at the front all day," another social worker said.

Suddenly I got serious. I cleared my throat a couple of times to get the Ground Zero crud out of my lungs and said, "Excuse me, ma'am, but the only thing that is bothering me is, when are they going to catch the assholes that bombed the Towers?"

Bill almost spit his coffee all over the room. He quickly recovered himself and said, "Well, if there is anything you want to talk about, don't hesitate to come to us," gesturing to the door and hoping that I would leave as soon as possible.

30
social worker

Weeks after the Trade Center crash things were still not back to normal.

The block party around the hospital was abruptly put to an end on the orders of one of the vice presidents of the hospital. The hospital was trying to get on with "business as usual," even though the rest of us were still reeling from the events.

The administration was trying to cut corners any way that they could think of. The hospital lost an awful lot of money treating patients for free and, when and if the federal funds arrived, the bookkeepers had to make up the money somehow. One of the first ways was to inform the medics that all the extra hours that they were putting in would be treated as straight time. They could not afford to pay us time-and-a-half. Hell, I would have volunteered for extra hours without pay.

But what really got the medics up in arms was a totally different matter.

There was an outpouring of material gratitude extended to the uniformed personnel of the city by major corporations and organizations, which became a source of low morale to noncity organizations. Nowhere was this exclusion felt more than by the paramedics of St. Vincent's Hospital. It was depressing to hear how FDNY personnel were given free vacations and cruises, free tickets to major sporting events and entertainment performances. There was a benefit concert at Madison Square Garden, hosted by major entertainment stars, not to mention free Broadway shows. None of us were invited.

It was more distressing to hear that FDNY and NYPD personnel who were nowhere near the Towers on the eleventh of September were the recipients of these gifts. It was not even the fact that we were not getting offered these gratuities, it was that we were not even being acknowledged for our contributions on 9/11. Quite frankly, I would have felt funny accepting these perks. I would rather they have been given to the families of the victims.

As with most problems in our ambulance department, we all sat around, bitching and complaining, and no one did anything about it.

Our hurt feelings were quickly replaced by anger when news was leaked that, among other things, tickets were issued for concerts and Broadway shows. It was rumored that there were also free passes to Disney World, gift certificates to the Gap clothing stores, vacations, and cruises. Although they were especially earmarked for the paramedics and emergency room doctors and nurses, the gifts were never seen by the rank and file.

The rumor mill painted a picture of persons unknown walking around with new clothes, taking free vacations, and going to see top entertainment and sporting events, including the World Series at Yankee Stadium.

When the news trickled down to the ambulance department, the only gifts that remained were passes to Disney World, which were to expire within the month. To my knowledge, only a couple of paramedics used the passes, since the expiration date quickly arrived.

With morale at it lowest and when just about all hope was lost for survivors, an hysterical woman came running into the hospital and said, "My husband just called me on his cell phone. He's a Port Authority police officer. He was inside the Towers when they collapsed!"

She went on and further explained, "He's with a group of other officers that are trapped inside a pocket in the basement, and they are still alive!"

"Still alive!" That was a phrase that no one ever thought they would hear.

In everybody's eagerness to believe her story, no one stopped to think that the cell phone batteries could not have lasted that long. Everyone jumped into action and all available hands went to the Pile and started digging. Most dug with their bare hands because there were not enough gloves available. They dug until their hands bled and then they dug some more.

The story was a hoax. This woman was not even married, and, besides causing mass confusion, she extended the hopes of the families who were already resolved to the fact that their loved ones were lost forever.

It was at about that time that I started to lose it. I had not released my sad emotions in any way. I, like others, was going deeper and deeper into a funk.

Shortly after the false alarm, one night, when I arrived at the hospital for my shift, my arms and legs started to get very weak. I did not have a clear thought in my head. Everything I attempted to do seemed very mechanical and disassociated. Gracie was my partner for the night and I could not hear a word she said. It really started to scare me.

After taking our first patient to the hospital, I found myself staring into space. As I stood in the Emergency Room, waiting to get triaged, I lost all focus of my surroundings and of time and space. This was it! I thought. This was the big one! I was going to end up a full-fledged EDP and be put in a pink gown reserved for crazy patients.

Suddenly, a middle-aged woman whom I had never seen before walked up to me. She touched my shoulder and started to speak: "Do you want to talk?"

I looked at her, confused. "Me?" I replied. She smiled and repeated her question in a softer voice. I nodded.

I do not remember much of what happened in the next few minutes, other than that I left Gracie with the patient. She was giving her report, and I found myself seated in a closed room with a stranger.

We talked for a while and I felt tears rolling down my cheeks. I did not get choked up at all, but the tears just kept flowing. This kind woman was a volunteer social worker and she saved my life that autumn night.

I began to realize that what was causing me to feel so badly was the fact that I did not help anyone who was under the rubble. I was also feeling terrible that I did not die on September 11. The question that I asked was the question so many others asked: "Why was I alive?"

Since I was not physically dead I was going to die inside, deep in my heart. I was not going to be alive again until others were found alive. Like so many, when all hope was finally lost, the

Towers finally came down on us, the survivors.

For a few people, coming apart at the seams happened quickly. Some people dealt with it when it happened. There was weeping and mourning right on the battlefield as soon as the Towers fell. For the majority, it did not happen until days and weeks after the crash.

What were we, the survivors, supposed to do? Quit our jobs? Some did, but most carried on and that is what I now hoped I could do.

The kind-hearted lady hugged me, thanked me for what I did, and told me that I would be alright. I really did not believe her, but I wanted to believe her. The migraine that I had developed made matters worse. Now I was in a fog and I could barely keep my eyes open from the pain in my forehead.

The night went on, the migraine subsided, and somehow by the grace of God my mind started to clear. As the 1,600 milligrams of Motrin started to kick in, it not only took away my headache but it opened my eyes to the world around me. The sun eventually came up on a new day.

I had a great gift—the gift of life, the gift of seeing another sunrise and enjoying the smell of a fresh-mown lawn. I also realized my responsibility to the honored dead. To live my life to the fullest and in the light of their supreme sacrifice. I was lucky enough to be walking the streets of Manhattan and enjoying the rain-soaked pavement. I was feeling the blood pumping through my veins and I had an infinite amount of possibilities. How many brave souls would love to trade places with me? I would carry on.

31

the big party

I received a very confusing telephone call one morning. It was from my supervisor, Bill Batista. I thought he was calling to ask me to cover a shift. We had a multitude of sick calls once autumn began. Everybody was sick and tired of being sick and tired.

"Frank. I'm calling to invite you to a party at the Waldorf Astoria," he said. "The hospital gives a dinner every year for its benefactors and this year they are inviting the medics of nine-eleven. You're going to be their guests of honor. The only catch was that you have to get a tuxedo."

Getting a tuxedo was no problem, since I still had one left over from my show business days. No. It was not a blue crushed velvet tuxedo. It had not been that long since I left the theater. Usually, I hated these kinds of affairs, but it would be worth it to see some of the other guys dressed up in formal wear.

When I arrived at the garage that night, I found out that many of the medics were disturbed about my invitation. It seems that not everyone was invited, only the five original crews.

"How did you and Carl get on the A-list?" asked Desmond Engle. "Most of the medics got to the city at around the same time you did. You didn't have the first Tower fall on you."

"We got to Ground Zero when the second building was

falling," I said.

It had become a real pissing match.

"Bill told me the medics of nine-eleven were being honored. I thought everyone was invited and that's why I accepted the invitation. Had I known that they were excluding anyone, I never would have said yes," I said.

"Nope, only the golden eight. I guess with you and Carl it's the platinum ten!" Desmond said, as some of the others in the garage laughed and others looked annoyed. The golden eight were the St. Vincent's paramedics who were on duty when the Towers first were hit.

"Look, if anybody would like to go in my place they can," I said.

One medic went as far as to say, "What did you do that was so special? I didn't see you here on the eleventh."

Bill Batista got irritated when he heard of this pettiness and explained to anybody that would listen, "Frank and Carl were in the first ambulance to arrive at the hospital and spent the next sixteen hours coming back and forth from the front."

He made it sound like it was a whole lot more than it was. But now, after what some of the medics had said, I was not in any mood to go to a party.

I later changed my mind since no one requested to go in my place; I thought it would be a waste to throw away a thousand-dollar-a-plate meal.

The meal was great. The master of ceremonies introduced the honored guests table by table. In the first table were representatives from the Sixth Precinct of the NYPD followed by members of FDNY's Squad 18. These are the precinct and firehouse in the vicinity of St. Vincent's. By the time they introduced the medics, the guests were applauding so loudly that

I doubt if anyone knew who the heck we were.

All in all the medics were cleaned up and looked as if they were at the Academy Awards. The only female medic who was part of the "platinum ten" was unable to attend, so as the night wore on and the alcohol started to flow, it became quite rowdy.

Some of the medics got really bagged up and started making a scene, commenting and cat-calling at the male and female opera singers. I am sure we wore out our welcome.

I had to leave early because I had an ambulance shift that night and needed to go change into my uniform. We were so short-staffed that I could not even get the night off. It was a blessing in disguise because I really wanted to get out of there.

32
another collapse

As I was eating the over-priced dinner, my partner Peter was in the middle of a brand new clusterfuck at Nineteenth Street and Park Avenue South, in the vicinity of Gramercy Park.

Scaffolding around a building renovation had collapsed, with all the construction workers either trapped or injured. Five workers would lose their lives and nearly a dozen more were injured. According to press reports most of the workers were underpaid Mexicans, which meant that not everything was being done according to code.

Peter and Kurt Schafer were called to the scene as well as Becky and another medic.

Being the first two units on the scene, the paramedics of St. Vincent's quickly took charge of the medical portion of the disaster. Peter and Kurt were awaiting extrication of patients. Anytime the firefighters and NYPD ESU cut away some debris, they would slide them to the medics for rapid evaluation and treatment.

Peter found a space in the rubble and quickly descended into the depths. He waited nearly two hours for the emergency workers to clear a path, and infused IV after IV to keep a trapped patient alive, using only the light from his flashlight to see.

another collapse

Becky helped Peter any way she could and tried more than once to change places, but he would not hear of it, in part because he did not want to leave his patient, not even for a second, but mainly because he did not want to put her in danger.

When the crew arrived at the hospital, I was waiting for them at the ambulance door. Still in my tuxedo, I helped them unload the last patient. Although the medics protested, because they were afraid to get my suit dirty, I hugged every last one of them. I was angry with myself that I was at that stupid dinner while they were out risking their lives. I really was tempted to do my shift in formal wear, but the supervisor would not approve my choice of clothing. So much for my night on the town.

33

everybody goes to Nino's

One of the best conditions supervisors in the City of New York is a medic named Harvey Costello. Harvey is a long-time member of EMS, and when it merged with FDNY he became one of its lieutenants. A conditions boss is an EMS lieutenant who supervises paramedic and EMT units in his assigned area. He is also in charge of all mass casualty incidents or calls that involve multiple patients. He is not in charge of patient care, only patient disposition and coordination of resources. The first paramedic unit on the scene is in charge of patient care.

Harvey usually works the night shift. He always cuts through the pettiness and just tries to lend a helping hand.

One night in early October, Peter and I were three blocks away from a quadruple shooting.

"Any municipal units in the vicinity of the Holland Tunnel?" the dispatcher asked.

The dispatcher repeated her question, but there was no response.

Suddenly the Nextel beeped.

"Are you guys listening to PD?" a voice queried.

"No. What's up?" Peter asked.

"It's Phil. Where are you guys?"

"At Varick and West Houston, getting coffee," Peter said.

"We're up at Roosevelt with a patient. You got a shooting at the tunnel."

Peter changed the channel on his radio and we heard PD frantically calling for a medic unit.

"Central. This is Zero Five William. Show us sixty-three to the Holland Tunnel," I said.

Peter put on the lights and sirens and we were on our way.

"Negative, Five Willie. Go to your eighty-nine."

Dispatch then tried to send an FDNY paramedic unit from uptown. Of course, Peter and I ignored the order and proceeded to the shooting, which was right outside the entrance of the Holland Tunnel.

"Central. This is Five William. Show us flagged at Varick and Broome Street by PD."

Several other units that were not officially dispatched to the location arrived shortly after we did. Since we were the first paramedic unit on the scene, we took charge of the situation and began triaging and treating the patients. Like us, the other units on the scene were monitoring the police department radio and proceeded to the Holland Tunnel before the EMS dispatcher sent out the call for help.

We found out later that this was some kind of drug deal gone bad.

Three young men were in a car at the mouth of the tunnel with unknown injuries. On our way to treat them we came upon another young man who had left his car for help. He had a gunshot wound to his leg and was lying on the ground writhing in pain and bleeding profusely.

"Don't worry, we're gonna fix you up," I said as I pulled out a trauma dressing from my medical bag.

"I'm going to see what's up with the other patients," Peter said as he ran towards the vehicle, not knowing whether or not the shooter was still at large.

Harvey Costello arrived on the scene and started coordinating patient care.

"You guys from Cabrini, take two of the patients in the car. Clare's will take the third patient and Vinny's got this one. Where do you want to go, Frankie?"

"Let's take them to Vinny's," I answered.

But the brass from FDNY and NYPD ordered us to Bellevue, a city hospital.

For all we knew, the FDR Drive would be packed and the streets were still impassable due to the events of September 11.

"This is my gig and these are my units. Follow us to St. Vincent's," said Harvey.

The FDNY and NYPD superior officers followed our caravan of four ambulances and a command car to St. Vincent's, arriving there in only a couple of minutes. Thankfully, all of the gunshot victims survived and were released shortly thereafter.

Near where the quadruple shooting took place was a restaurant called Nino's. Nino's was located on Canal Street at the foot of the Ground Zero roadblocks. I do not really know who Nino was, but the owner decided to close down his restaurant to the public on September 11. However, he opened his doors to all of the Ground Zero workers and the regular police, firefighters, and emergency medical service workers of Lower Manhattan.

Nino's restaurant had been open twenty-four hours a day, seven days a week, since the beginning of the crisis. With food donated from various sources and an army of volunteers, the restaurant served meals and snacks at any time of the day or night. Also, local entertainers performed in the restaurant as emergency workers devoured meal after meal. It was a haven from the devastation and depression of the conditions we had to endure long after the cameras left and the hoopla died down.

Harvey was the crown prince of Nino's. He would hold court every night with his men and make sure all of us got a hot meal or a cup of coffee at sometime during the long overnight shift. Harvey must have gained thirty pounds since Nino's starting serving meals. His uniform jacket looker tighter and tighter every time we saw him. As much as his time was spent in the restaurant, he never once missed a call or compromised his duty. He was just trying to make an unbearable situation bearable. He succeeded.

In the hearts and minds of the workers, Nino's will never be forgotten. The firefighters, police, paramedics, EMTs, rescue workers, and volunteers had a common bond. Everybody went to Nino's.

Later on that night, Peter and I went to Nino's and we were greeted by Harvey. We sat down and had some hot soup and a soda at Harvey's table. Harvey spoke to both of us.

"We're probably gonna get jammed-up by Dispatch," said Peter.

"You probably won't be so popular with the brass," I said to Harvey.

"When the shit hits the fan, I want all available paramedics on scene. If there are too many of them, I'll reassign them. Not Dispatch. Don't worry about Dispatch. I'll handle Dispatch."

As we sat there I noticed that all of us were getting a little tight around the waist.

Sadly, Nino's closed its doors permanently a few months later, a victim of poor business conditions in Lower Manhattan after 9/11.

34
thanksgiving

In November, the days and weeks finally started to pass
quickly. Manhattanites went back to their normal annoying
behavior. Again they were complaining about the noise that our
ambulances made and the smell from the exhaust. Cabbies
once more were happily cutting us off at every opportunity.
But there was a different feeling throughout the city.

The normal hustle and bustle of Christmas shoppers was
noticeably absent. It was probably because some shoppers
were afraid to come into the city. I also think that people were
generally depressed because of the grim events. However,
there was a mass pilgrimage to Ground Zero, as it became the
newest tourist attraction.

Peter and I worked Five William, tour-one on Thanksgiving
morning. It was relatively quiet, except for the occasional drunk.
It was rumored that Nino's was serving a full turkey dinner, and
even the great chef Emeril Lagasse was making an appearance
to cook the rescue workers a gourmet meal.

We were both nodding off when a call came in.

"Zero Five William," the dispatcher called.

"Five Willie," Peter answered.

"Five William, proceed to Twenty-one and Eight for the inbleed."

"Send it over, Central," Peter replied.

As I copied the information sent by Central Dispatch from the KDT, the onboard computer, I groused, "Great. An inbleed in the projects."

We both thought it was going to be pretty much bullshit, but we rushed to the scene nonetheless. On the elevator the smell of old urine and bug spray burned our nostrils. In the hallway outside the patient's apartment, a young Hispanic woman greeted us.

"Hurry up, yo. My uncle has the seizures and he's spitting up blood. Hurry. Hurry."

"Does he have a history of seizures?" Peter inquired.

"Yes. But he is really spitting up a lot of blood."

Seizures? But where is the blood coming from? Probably he bit his tongue, we both thought.

Peter and I walked past two police officers who were in the doorway and saw an older man lying on the floor in a pool of liquid with thick blood on his chin, mouth, and chest. This was no tongue bleed. He was pale and looking as if he was on death's door. He was barely conscious and moaning loudly. While Peter was getting a quick history from the family members, I was doing a rapid assessment.

"Pete. I can't get a pulse," I explained, as I pressed my fingers at first on his wrist and then near his Adam's apple.

I could not get a pulse in his carotid artery, which meant his systolic blood pressure was less than 60. This guy was about to crap out.

"It looks as if he's got esophageal varices," Peter barked at me as he put away the paperwork and tossed me an IV start-pack. He began opening one for himself. Basically, esophageal varices are tears in the tube leading down to the stomach, and there can be massive bleeding involved. I never saw this condition before, but I trusted Peter implicitly. He would always clarify any medical questions I had and was a great diagnostician. I tried to do my share as a partner by trying to be a competent clinician. We were always learning from one another.

It also looked as if the patient was bleeding out of both ends because his bottom was covered with blood. He had lost, at the very least, a liter of blood. I started to spike an IV bag while Peter tried to get a line on his right arm.

The two police officers stood in horror as we tried desperately to find a vein.

"Do you guys need any help?" one of the officers asked.

Usually we would give them a "fifty–five" which means they were free to leave.

"Can you guys stick around for a couple of minutes? We could probably use your help in another minute," Peter said.

The only vein Peter could find blew immediately because the patient's vasculature was so compromised. I tossed Peter another IV bag as I stomped on the cockroaches that covered the floor. I searched for a vein in the man's other arm. It was pretty hopeless. His arm was scarred, probably from IV drug use in his youth, and his skin was thick as leather. I saw a small vein in the inside part of his wrist and was able to pass a small needle. We quickly infused the man with IV fluids and loaded him on the stretcher with the help of the two police officers.

Peter thought quickly and immediately moved the man into the shock position, which probably saved his life. Many times paramedics forget what they learned as EMTs, which is basic first aid. We get so caught up in pushing drugs that we forget that basic life support is as important as advanced life support. "BLS before ALS," is a saying that is drilled into your head throughout medic school. The simple act of raising a patient's legs and warming the body is sometimes as effective as giving a life-saving drug.

By the time we got the patient into the ambulance I was able to feel a pulse in his neck and his vital signs approached normal levels. When we got him to the hospital he stopped moaning and was becoming more and more alert. Quick treatment by the Emergency Department staff at St. Vincent's helped this man to live another day.

"You saved his life," said Doctor Stanley Sturgis as he passed us.

"No, Pete saved his life," I said.

"No, you saved his life," said Peter.

This went back and forth a couple of times as I wrote up the paperwork and Peter cleaned the stretcher. This was our regular routine.

As the night came to an end, the man who was near death was sitting up in bed and talking to his loved ones. What could have been a painful memory in the lives of his family became a real source of Thanksgiving.

35
new year's eve

New Year's Eve started out pretty slowly and the mood felt somber. That was partly due to the heightened security in anticipation of another terrorist attack that night. Because of the events of 9/11, Peter and I did not feel much like celebrating, which is why we volunteered for the holiday tour. Also, we wanted to be on the job if the shit hit the fan.

"Zero Five Willie, respond to Thirty-second and Seven for the stab," the radio sounded.

Peter and I drove uptown, and when we arrived there were several RMPs and a large group of Asian men arguing over something. The police barely noticed our presence. There was no stabbing, just a lot of men with high testosterone levels.

The police just waved us past.

"This is going to be a ten-ninety, Central. Police matter only. They don't need us yet," I radioed to Central Dispatch.

Peter and I grabbed a quick cup of coffee and decided to head for one of our usual spots on Bleeker Street and MacDougal to watch the parade of party-goers.

As we sat there we saw an RMP from the Sixth Precinct barrel past us with the emergency lights on.

"What the hell is going on?" I said.

"Put on PD radio," Peter said.

"Let's get behind them," I said, as I adjusted my radio to listen to the police frequency.

The police frequency was buzzing with a call for shots fired on the Lower East Side. I immediately punched in our status as ninety–eight on the KDT. That tells the dispatcher that we are no longer at our eighty–nine but are available for a job within our battalion. I did this so we could buff the job.

As Peter and I proceeded to First Avenue where the shooting was supposed to be, we heard the paramedics on Seven King come over the radio.

"Tell all units to stay out of the area. Shots fired!"

The first thought I had was "scene safety." This was quickly replaced by my concern for the crew of Seven King. "What the hell is the deal? Are they under fire? Screw scene safety!"

Peter and I were now a block away from where the shots were supposed to have happened when I got on the radio. "Zero Five William. Put us on Seven King's back. We're a block away from First Avenue and East Seven Street."

"Remain ninety–eight Five William. No ALS needed at this time," the dispatcher replied.

Peter and I continued to go to the scene and find out what was happening.

When we arrived we saw two plain-clothes police officers covering the body of a young man in his twenties. He was obviously bleeding. Other police officers were waving us on.

The young man had been in an altercation with another man and had been shot in the process. The shooter was now in a bar across the street holding eight people hostage. He poured gasoline over his hostages and was threatening to blow them up.

Peter and I were now caught in a crossfire between the police and the shooter.

When Peter stopped the ambulance, shots were being fired at my side of the ambulance. Peter quickly got out of the ambulance and started to do a modified low crawl. I hopped over to his side of the ambulance and followed him out. It was just as if we were back in the Marine Corps on routine infantry maneuvers.

We both made patient contact and I stayed with the patient while Peter went for the stretcher. I started to drag the patient towards the ambulance and Peter met me halfway there with the stretcher. With the help of the two police officers, one of whom was bleeding from the hand, we moved the patient to the stretcher and then into our ambulance as shots rang out around us.

Just then a conditions boss ran up to our ambulance.

"What the fuck are you doing here? You were told to stay back."

"We were getting our patient," I said.

"We have a fucking BLS unit on the way."

"Hey Lieutenant, calm your ass down. We have the patient now," Peter said as we quickly started an IV line and treated the patient for shock.

"He has no pulse," I yelled to Peter as I felt the patient's wrist and neck.

"Wait for the fucking BLS unit. That's an order!"

"You gotta be fucking shitting me?" Peter exclaimed.

"I don't appreciate your cursing at me," the conditions boss said.

Peter and I always do the good cop, bad cop routine. Sometimes, however, it becomes bad cop, horrible cop.

"Hey Lieutenant, either hop on the bus and give us a hand or get the fuck out of here!" I shouted.

The BLS unit arrived as Peter ran to the front of the ambulance to drive to the hospital. It was an FDNY-EMT unit that covers part of the Lower East Side of Manhattan. One of the EMTs was a student in the St. Vincent's paramedic program, the other was Joe McArthur, a veteran EMT.

"What have you got, Frankie?" McArthur asked.

"We got one patient with a GSW (gunshot wound). There's also a cop who got shot in the hand."

"You take the cop, Joe," I ordered.

"You got it," McArthur replied, seeing that we had our patient ready to go and that I was about to start a second IV line.

"Ready, partner?" Peter shouted from the front of the ambulance.

"Hold it," the conditions boss screamed. "Let Four Henry take the GSW."

"Move it out, Peter," I yelled. I slammed the door and watched as the conditions boss's face got red with rage. I also saw the EMTs give me a tip of their caps in approval as they hurried the police officer into their ambulance. As first paramedics on scene, we were in charge of patient care.

The conditions boss ran to the front of the ambulance and yelled to Peter, "You're not taking him to Vinny's!"

Peter yelled back, "Of course not, you moron!"

From the time we made patient contact until the patient was in the trauma room of Bellevue Hospital, a period of only twelve minutes elapsed. The young man was shot twice, once to the abdomen and once to the chest. His bleeding was stopped and his wounds sealed. He received more than a liter of fluid via two large bore IVs. He went from having no pulse to having a normal pulse rate and blood pressure en route to the hospital. He was taken up to the operating room and had a full recovery.

The hostages were later freed when the police stormed the building. The hostage taker was shot and wounded, but he also survived.

After leaving Bellevue, before we could get back to our eighty–nine, we received a call for a male on the tracks at Penn Station.

When we arrived at the underground police station we found a man in his forties with an open compound fracture. Bones were protruding from his ankle and there was a moderate amount of blood. It did not seem that there was an artery involved because the blood was not spurting out. The patient had been taken from the tracks and brought to the precinct office. He had alcohol on his breath, as did a buddy. They were both dressed in the clothes of civilian workers of Ground Zero. It seems that after work the two men got drunk and one of them stumbled onto the tracks. Normally, we would have thought that the two men were idiots for being so careless, but after months at the Pile, their intoxication was probably well-deserved, so we treated them with a lot more understanding, knowing the stress they were under.

Quickly, we stabilized the leg and stopped the residual bleeding. We put the man on a long board and cervical collar, and along with the help of a few police officers, we carried him up the stairs and into the ambulance.

We drove him to the closest hospital, where the surgical team was alerted, and he was taken to the trauma room to receive more definitive treatment. As we restocked our supplies and wrote up the paperwork, we saw Carl come up to us, shaking his head in disbelief and looking as if he was anxious to tell us the latest gossip.

"They dropped him," he said. "They dropped him right on his bad leg."

The ER staff forgot to put up the safety bar on the bed. Our patient must have moved and rolled off the bed and hit the floor.

Now the poor bastard probably had a worse trauma than when we brought him in. Luckily, he was too drunk to feel any pain and, miraculously, it did not complicate his leg problems. Unbelievably, he was released the next day after surgery.

As we walked out of the hospital, pushing the stretcher, I turned to Peter, who asked, "Chicken legs?"

"I was thinking more about Buffalo wings, if we can find a place that's open," I replied.

One of the strangest things that Peter and I do is related to food. We have food desensitization therapy after every disgusting call. It is our way of being able to eat certain foods without gagging. Here's how it works. In the case of seeing a patient with an open fracture, we go and eat chicken wings. One of the reasons is, if we do not eat something similar to what we just saw on the ambulance call, one day we will be sitting at the dinner table with our families and we will gag when thinking of a previous disgusting mental picture.

If we treat a patient who throws up, we will immediately go to a restaurant and eat split pea soup. A burn patient usually means that we will be eating barbequed ribs. A snotty-nosed patient requires us to eat vegetable chow mein.

We once had a patient who was morbidly obese. The skin was bumpy and gray in color. We ate oatmeal that morning for breakfast because it was the food that most resembled the thing that almost made us sick. It was difficult to get the food down, but I can still eat oatmeal and not be sceeved out. Now we can eat just about anything at any time without loss of appetite, no matter how nasty an ambulance call may have been.

36

the new year

Thank God there were no terrorist attacks on New Year's Eve as so many people had anticipated. The new year had a surprise in store of a different kind.

Back in October we received word that Ronald Reagan, king of the bums, had died at Bellevue Hospital. The male indigent community was distraught and many of them, despite their sadness, vied for the vacant position. I, too, felt sorry, because Ronald was a familiar character and, after all, he was a human being and did have a place in the life of the streets.

"Doesn't it make you a little sad?" I asked Peter.

Peter just looked at me and furrowed his brow, "Why? He was a pain in the ass. He didn't contribute a damn thing other than soaking the taxpayers of their hard-earned money. He was an annoying, smelly skell."

Still, I wondered how a person could get to the point of no return: he was a complete sociopath, who could not hold a job, had no home or could not maintain any real caring relationships. How do people get that far away from the mainstream?

Late in January, I was passing Fourteenth Street and Eighth Avenue on the overnight tour and I saw a middle-aged man with white hair and a new coat. His hair was somewhat matted, but he was clean-shaven. I remarked to my rookie partner Charles,

"Look, a new Ronald Reagan." We both chuckled.

As we drew nearer to the corner, I realized that it was not a new Ronald Reagan. It was Ronald Reagan, back from the dead once again. I got on the Nextel phone and called the other units. No one believed me, especially Peter, when I told him the next day.

Weeks passed, and then, one morning while Peter and I were sitting in front of the ER in our ambulance, I saw Carl and one of the other medics wheeling in a patient. They both looked at me angrily and I could not understand why. After taking the patient into the hospital, they both approached my ambulance.

"You wished him back to life. It's your fault," Carl said.

"Ronald Reagan? It didn't even look like him," I said.

"It's him. Believe me, you couldn't miss his brand of stink."

"See, Pete. I told you," I said.

Peter just shook his head in disbelief as the radio sounded.

"Five William. Two-four and Eight for the respiratory arrest: twenty-three-year-old female not breathing, possible overdose."

epilogue

other units involved in the 9/11 rescues

Seven King

On the morning of the crash, paramedics Diego Rodriguez and Roberta "Bobbie" Pederson had staffed Seven King and were working as EMTs.

Diego parked his ambulance in the shadow of the North Tower and he and Bobbie treated the many burned and injured patients that hurried towards them.

While they were in the thick of aiding people, pieces of the North Tower fell off, pelting Diego and Bobbie with debris. In the confusion, Bobbie ran three blocks north, leaving her partner temporarily behind. Once the shower of junk subsided, Diego continued to treat the injured alone, and Bobbie rejoined him at the corner of Church and Vesey Streets.

They treated patients until their supplies were almost spent, then they loaded up their vehicle with patients and proceeded north to St. Vincent's Hospital, but Diego stopped partway and discharged them because they were all ambulatory. They could continue to the hospital on foot.

His duty was to take only patients that could *not* walk,

otherwise the lame would be left behind.

Diego and Bobbie then drove back into the hot zone and set up a new triage center somewhere near West Broadway and Murray Street. Again, they started to treat the walking wounded and helped those that could not walk onto the ambulance, when the second plane hit making the South Tower explode into flames.

When the last patients were loaded into the ambulance, Diego manipulated his vehicle forward while it started to get struck with falling debris. Panic-stricken people began to jump onto the running boards on the sides and back of the ambulance, causing him to proceed slowly and calmly in spite of the safety risk.

By the Grace of God, Seven King made it out of the oven with the passengers and patients unharmed. Diego and Bobbie's courage, self-discipline, tenacity, and devotion to duty saved many lives.

Three Victor

The second St. Vincent's unit to arrive at the Towers was Three Victor, tour two, staffed by Gary Chester and Esteban Guerrero. After hearing that a plane had crashed into one of the Towers, they raced to the scene and found thousands of people filling the streets.

Esteban quickly deployed his vehicle a few blocks away from the Towers under a pedestrian bridge near building Number Six.

The two medics got out and surveyed the scene. Dozens of people rushed towards the ambulance, demanding to be treated.

Chester and Esteban continued to treat patients, taking precautions not to load their ambulance beyond its capacity. They brought a half-dozen people to the hospital and treated many more at the scene.

Later that morning they made another attempt to go down to the crash site. Arriving at the AMEX building, shortly after the South Tower collapsed, they were forced to retreat from the building with a load of patients when it was feared that it would also collapse.

Five William

Earlier, Ned Edwards and Andrew Johns had replaced Peter and me on Five William in ambulance 1778. After eating breakfast they pulled their vehicle in front of the hospital and were immediately sent to treat a patient having a severe asthma attack. After spending a half hour on scene, stabilizing and packaging the patient, they were transporting the individual to St. Vincent's when Ned heard an extensive series of numbers on the radio.

As they arrived at the hospital, two ER doctors were standing in front of the hospital with a large group of hospital personnel. They all faced south and looked in horror.

"What is going on?" asked Andrew.

"A plane crashed into the Towers about two minutes ago," a young doctor said.

After setting their patient inside, they traveled down Seventh Avenue and West Street and immediately began treating patients at the MERV that was set up by FDNY-EMS, adjacent to the

epilogue

Towers on Chambers and West Streets.

Debris was falling on top of them from the crashed plane. Andrew looked up and saw objects floating to the ground, which looked like large birds.

"Look at the size of those birds," he remarked.

They got larger and larger as they came to the ground. As they fell around him, just missing him at times, he realized that the birds were in fact human beings.

People hurried over to the mobile hospital to be helped and healed. Although there were wounded police officers and firefighters, most of the casualties were civilian.

When a second plane crashed into the South Tower, glass shards and debris were showered down upon the MERV. Ned and Andrew, along with others in the area, had to run for their lives. Heading in opposite directions, as they began to get pelted with more and more debris, Andrew crawled under the MERV, grabbing several patients who were unable to walk. Ned and the others tried to outrun the oncoming wave of wreckage.

After the initial debris fell, Ned tried to make his way back to the ambulance in order to ready the vehicle to transport the mounting casualties. He never actually got there. Instead, he retrieved his medical bag from the MERV and started looking for patients to treat. More and more debris started falling, and finally vehicle 1778 was covered with rubble.

Amid the chaos, Andrew continued to treat patients at the MERV, but had to run for his life again when suddenly, and without warning, the South Tower collapsed to the ground.

Ned, who was in the same area, again tried to outrun the falling wreckage. He made it as far as the railing that bordered the Hudson River and was about to take a leap into the water when, fortunately, the oncoming debris stopped short.

Andrew treated firefighters and civilians where he stood. As the air filled with smoke and dust he fought desperately to breathe and to see.

Miraculously, Ned led patients back to other ambulances, but not before making several other attempts to get back to his own vehicle and find Andrew. When Ned finally got to the spot where his ambulance once stood, it was gone. Someone had either moved it or it was now completely covered with debris. He met up with conditions boss Harvey Costello, and took a few critically injured patients back to St. Vincent's in an SUV.

Thankfully, Andrew made it back to the hospital later that day.

Javits Center Medics

The State of New York operates the Jacob K. Javits Convention Center, and St. Vincent's Hospital has a contract with the state to provide medical care in the form of paramedics, nurses, and doctors.

On the morning of the eleventh Paulie Caravella and Daniel Hughes were scheduled to work the Javits tour.

They arrived at the garage around nine a.m., shortly after the first tower was hit.

As they loaded their ambulance at the West Street garage, ready to head south, two men entered the building. One was a police officer, the other was a civilian holding his leg. Paulie saw that it was an open compound fracture.

Paulie and Daniel raced north on West Street with their patient, who was in severe distress. The veteran paramedics rapidly stabilized his injury while they rushed him to the hospital. As they drove to St. Vincent's a call came over the radio that a second plane had hit the South Tower. In disbelief they anxiously continued to the Emergency Room with their potentially unstable patient.

The two medics then hurried back to their ambulance, then headed south with lights and sirens blaring. When they arrived at the crash site, the two Towers were still standing and they quickly went to work.

"You set up here. I'm going over by the American Express building," said Daniel.

"Don't lose sight of the bus," Paulie cautioned his partner.

At one time, St. Vincent's had a medic unit stationed in the World Trade Center, but that was many years before. Daniel had decades of experience as a medic and was a veteran of the old Trade Center unit, so he knew the area very well, including the ins and outs of the surrounding buildings. Daniel remembered that there was a nursing home nearby and headed to it on foot.

Daniel found a path to the nursing home, and after making sure that the patients were being evacuated—most of them were not ambulatory—he made his way back to the Towers just as the first building was falling.

People were shouting, "The building is falling! The building is falling!"

"Follow me. I know a way out," Daniel ordered, as he led a mass exodus through the American Express building, glass shards showering the lobby.

While Daniel was helping people escape, Paulie continued treating people on the street. He took care of their wounds until his medical bag was empty. He felt sickened when he saw the Towers fall and he did not know the whereabouts of his old friend Daniel.

Meanwhile, Daniel got his followers several blocks south of the Towers, near Liberty Street. It was his knowledge of the buildings that allowed him to save so many lives that day, while barely escaping with his own.

Other Units

Emergency units from all over the metropolitan area came pouring in to help for the anticipated thousands of casualties. Staging areas were set up throughout Lower Manhattan, especially at the Chelsea Piers, on West Street and on Twenty-third. Ambulances from New Jersey, Long Island, Connecticut, and upstate New York supplemented FDNY and New York hospital-based ambulances ready to relieve the units up on the line.

In the days to follow units as far away as California and Canada joined the ranks of rescue workers. These were the best and the finest that our nation and continent had to offer. These out-of-town men and women became New Yorkers by adoption, baptized by the tears and blood that they had shed saving our city.

afterword

Many months have passed since that hot day in September of 2001. Thankfully, our city has started to heal. The bravery of the paramedics, EMTs, fire department, police, and other emergency workers continues.

Incredibly, not one St. Vincent's paramedic has left the job. I attribute this to our devotion to our city and the support of our hospital. A dozen new paramedics have been added to our ranks and the work continues.

Most of the "golden eight" are still manning the daytime shift at St. Vincent's.

My regular partners Gracie, Carl, and Peter are still serving as street doctors. Carl, no longer a rookie, is now the grand old man of the night shift, having more experience than the majority of nighttime paramedics. Gracie is going for her master's degree in teaching while raising a family and working full-time. Powder became a good friend on our regular Friday-night shifts together. Peter left the "dark side" and is now a daytime paramedic. He is happily running five miles a day, keeping regular hours, and is salty as ever.

In the year that followed the attack on our soil, my life surely changed. I grew to have a different understanding and respect for the people I call my family and friends.

afterword

Right after Peter left Five William, I was appointed paramedic supervisor. After several failed attempts to enlist in the military, I resolved that my place to serve was at St. Vincent's Hospital in the City of New York. I served in that capacity until the beginning of 2003. It was an honor to be a supervisor for the men and women who served so bravely at the Towers and continue to serve everyday as unsung heroes.

I have many blessings that many people who were affected by the tragedy could not count as theirs. First and foremost, I am alive and so are my partners. I have two beautiful daughters who are growing up to be the kind of people who care for others. They have a mother who is teaching them to be good women. I am blessed to have Tammy in my life now and in the future.

Although I am no longer a supervisor, I continue to work as a paramedic at St. Vincent's and continue to write.

appendix

paramedics and New York City EMS

While I have changed the unit designations for the purposes of this book, the regular units for St. Vincent's Hospital are Seven William, Two Victor, Six King, and the Javits Center. During the World Trade Center crisis the enhancement units put into service, Fifty-one William, Fifty-one X–ray, and finally, Sixty Victor, were manned by St. Vincent's paramedics.

Six King is the Basic Life Support unit operated by St. Vincent's Paramedics. Usually EMTs operate a BLS unit, but since St. Vincent's does not employ EMTs, paramedics make up the crew of Six King, although the crew can only function as EMTs. While on Six King they carry no drugs except oxygen and epinephrine for patients who are having a severe allergic reaction. By law, they are not allowed to use their paramedic skills while on duty. Six King does not have a regular crew. In a given two-week period, full-time paramedics work seven shifts on an ALS unit and on the Six King BLS unit for three shifts.

Units are designated more or less according to their sector. The number designates the geographical sector. The letter indicates whether or not the unit is ALS or BLS. The 911 system uses the phonetic alphabet. 03V would be Zero Two Victor or Two Victor for short. The upper half of the alphabet, usually letters A-M, is for BLS units, while the lower half, usually letters T-Z, is reserved for ALS units. Thus 03A would be Zero Three Adam and this would be a BLS unit in Sector or Battalion Three.

When the public dials 911, it will get an emergency vehicle that corresponds to the seriousness of the emergency. If the 911 operator classifies a patient as sick, a Basic Life Support ambulance staffed by EMTs will respond. On the other hand, if they classify a patient as having chest pain or some other imminently life-threatening condition, an ALS ambulance staffed by paramedics who can perform advanced interventions will go.

In most cases an EMT is the first contact that the public has with the EMS. EMTs have more patient contact, by far, than paramedics, and most times they have to be better diagnosticians than paramedics. Paramedics know that every call they get sent on is potentially a life-threatening call. EMTs have to be able to discern whether or not to treat the patient on their own or to call for paramedics. In most cases EMTs treat minor medical problems and traumas.

When you start working in the emergency medical service, the first thing you are taught, and the one thing that is drilled into your head most of all is "scene safety." Is the scene safe? If not, wait until police or firefighters secure it. Medics and EMTs are non-combatants. If we die, there is no one to take care of the wounded. We become part of the problem instead of part of the solution. We have to live so we can help the injured and sick.

Emergency Medical Technicians are pre-hospital medical personnel with about 125 hours of medical training in basic life support and first aid. They are allowed to use an automatic external defibrillator for patients in cardiac arrest.

Paramedics are highly skilled medical personnel with an additional 1,500 to 2,000 hours of medical training in a variety of adult and pediatric advanced life support interventions. To put it into perspective, let's take a look at a doctor's knowledge. Doctors go to school for four years after college and spend additional years in specialty training as interns and residents. Paramedics follow a two-year curriculum which, for most, is crammed into one year.

Doctors have a knowledge base of about sixty percent of medicine. Out of that sixty percent they are generally required to recall about twenty percent from memory. A paramedic has to know about fifteen percent of what a doctor knows. However, out of that fifteen percent, paramedics have to recall one hundred percent from memory.

Paramedics have to know more about emergency medicine and advanced cardiac life support than some doctors. For better or for worse, paramedics are "street doctors."

The training required for paramedics is equivalent to approximately two years of college. It consists of course work in adult and pediatric advanced cardiac life support, advanced CPR, and advanced traumatic life support. Courses are taken in anatomy and physiology, pharmacology, pathophysiology, airway management, routine and acute physical examination, treatment of hemorrhage and shock, head injuries, musculoskeletal trauma, head and spinal trauma, abdominal and thoracic trauma, toxicology, hazardous materials, burns, mass casualty incidents, cardiology, obstetrics, gynecology, and pediatric emergencies. The paramedic is also trained to treat most types of medical emergencies.

Because of their knowledge of pharmacology, paramedics have a variety of drugs at their disposal, including narcotics.

In the field and on the ambulance, a paramedic is able to treat most emergencies as effectively as in an emergency room. That is why, in most cases, a team of paramedics treats a patient on scene rather that rushing to a hospital. Definitive treatment can be given in the field and a patient's life can be saved, or his or her condition stabilized, before transport. Usually, transport is one of the last options of a paramedic crew.

Paramedics routinely treat all cardiac emergency by both electrical and drug therapy. They treat asthma, emphysema and other respiratory emergencies, traumas of all kinds, obstetric emergencies, and childbirth. Medics in the field commonly treat allergic reactions and drug overdoses.

Unlike other medical professionals, New York City paramedics are required to take the state and city certification exams every three years, and most opt to take the National Registry exam.

In New York City 911 paramedics and EMTs are either hospital-based or work for the FDNY. Both are sent to 911 calls and both operate under the same medical protocols. The Bureau of Emergency Medical Service is a strange setup. New York City EMS was once under the control of the Health & Hospitals Corporation. During the Rudolph Giuliani administration EMS was taken over by the Fire Department.

What it means today is that the emergency medical technicians and paramedics who work for the Fire Department ride on ambulances that have the FDNY logo on them. They also wear uniforms resembling firefighters except they have "EMT" or "Paramedic" on their shirts instead of the embroidered "FDNY." FDNY–EMTs and paramedics have a different pay scale and work schedule than do firefighters. They do not share firehouses or have the same benefits as firefighters.

Prior to 9/11 the city decided to downsize all emergency services. The Giuliani administration came up with the idea of sending firefighters to medical calls by making firefighters "first responders." First responders are trained in first aid and oxygen administration, which is below the EMT—basic level. By doing this, he created an additional duty for firefighters, thus saving many of their jobs.

When a 911 operator receives a medical call, firefighters are dispatched first, and then the call goes out to EMTs and/or paramedics on a separate radio frequency.

Conditions bosses, lieutenants of FDNY-EMS, handle supervision of all units in the 911 system. Central Dispatch, commanded by captains and above, assigns units to a call, but on the street the conditions lieutenants are in charge.

FDNY-EMS handles only a portion of the 911 calls in the five boroughs of New York. Although FDNY-EMS officers supervise all EMS personnel, the 911 calls are also handled by the "voluntary hospitals." Voluntary hospitals encompass all noncity-owned hospitals that volunteer to participate in the 911 system.

Paramedics and EMTs who work for voluntary hospitals are paid by the hospitals. Voluntary hospitals attempt to recoup their costs by billing their patients for medical services performed on the ambulances as well as the cost of transportation to the hospitals.

The main mission of the hospital-based units is patient care and transport. In addition to the above, FDNY-EMS is responsible for incident scene safety, MCIs, MEDEVACS (medical evacuations), HAZMATS (hazardous materials), fires and crimes in progress, and unusual public health or safety emergencies.

Since the voluntary hospital ambulances are technically New York City ambulances, they do not automatically take patients to their sponsoring hospital. They are required to take patients to the hospital of their choice, within reason. For instance, if a St. Clare's ambulance gets a 911 call and the patient asks to go to Bellevue, a city-owned hospital, the ambulance crew cannot take the patient to St. Clare's. The only time a crew makes a decision to take a patient to a hospital of the crew's choice is if that patient needs immediate care and the patient's hospital choice is farther away.

Most of the general public has no idea how the system works. Most do not know the difference between an EMT and a paramedic, let alone an FDNY ambulance and a voluntary hospital ambulance. Many people think FDNY ambulance crews are firemen and that voluntary ambulance crews work for private companies.

There are two types of ambulances in the New York City EMS system. The Basic Life Support ambulances are each staffed by two emergency medical technicians. Two paramedics staff each Advanced Life Support ambulance. Depending upon the severity of the emergency, a basic or advanced life support ambulance is dispatched.

When a St. Vincent's paramedic ambulance pulls up to a house some people think that we are a private transport ambulance. Some people also think that we are trying to shanghai them to St. Vincent's. Neither is true. If we suggest that they go to St. Vincent's it is because it is the nearest hospital in most cases, but we never take a patient there against his or her will.

The majority of paramedics in Lower Manhattan are hospital-based, not FDNY-EMS.

glossary

AED. Automatic External Defibrillator. A portable electronic device carried by EMTs that restores a normal rhythm to a patient's heart in cardiac arrest. It does not jumpstart a heart. It only works if there is certain electronic activity still present.

ALS. Advanced Life Support. Synonymous with paramedicine. Emergency medical treatments involving drug and advanced electronic therapy.

ALS AMBULANCE. In New York City two paramedics staff an Advanced Life Support ambulance.

BEMS. Pronounced bee-miss. Bureau of Emergency Medical Services, a branch of FDNY. Synonymous with FDNY-EMS. Hospital–based EMS units are FDNY–participating 911 ambulances. FDNY–EMS and hospital based units are dispatched to emergency calls in New York City when citizens dial 911.

BLS. Basic Life Support. First aid, cardiopulmonary resuscitation and oxygen therapy.

BLS AMBULANCE. In New York City, Basic Life Support ambulances are staffed by two emergency medical technicians.

BOLUS. A measured dose of a drug.

BUS. Another name for an ambulance.

BUFF. Buff can be used as a noun or a verb. When used to describe a medic, a "buff" is a person who is a wannabe EMS worker. EMS is like a hobby for buffs, and they collect any and all paraphernalia. They also have sirens and lights in their personal cars and have the latest and most trendy equipment and uniforms. To buff a call is to go to an unassigned ambulance call. To buff a job is to show you are being a hard-charging medic or EMT. Nobody likes a buff, but everybody likes to buff!

CARDIAC MONITOR. A lifepack. A portable device that is similar to an AED, but that has advanced functions such as those used in a hospital emergency room. A paramedic selects the settings manually. It can be used for defibrillation, cardioversion, and external pacing. It can also record electrocardiograms.

DISCRETIONARY ORDERS. Medical and pharmacological treatments not covered in a paramedic's protocol standing orders or medical control options. They must be authorized by telemetry. For example: giving a medication for an illness or injury not included in the protocols, such as giving morphine for noncardiac related pain. There is no general pain protocol for paramedic treatments.

EDP. Emotionally Disturbed Person. Referred to sometimes as "Every Day Person."

EMS. Emergency Medical Services.

EMT or **EMT-D.** Emergency Medical Technician. A health professional trained in basic life support and cardiac defibrillation using an AED.

ESU. Emergency Services Unit of the New York City Police and Corrections departments. These units are trained in special tactics and also emergency medical response. All ESU officers are also EMTs and some are paramedics.

FDNY. Pronounced fid-nee. Abbreviation for the Fire Department of New York.

HOSPITAL 02. Bellevue Hospital, Manhattan.

HOSPITAL 21. Saint Vincent's Hospital, Manhattan.

MANDATION. When a medic or EMT is required to work an extra eight hours after a relief calls in sick.

MCI. Mass Casualty Incident. An incident where five or more people are injured.

MEDICAL CONTROL OPTIONS. Treatments given to patients that are in protocol, but not part of a paramedic's standing orders. For example: giving a patient a sodium bicarbonate injection who is in asystolic cardiac arrest. It is used especially for an order to give narcotics or extra doses of drugs given on standing orders.

MERV. A Mobile Emergency Response Vehicle; a kind of mobile hospital.

MOS. Member of Service; uniformed personnel.

MUNICIPAL UNITS. ALS and BLS ambulances that are operated by New York City and staffed by FDNY-EMS personnel.

NRB. Nonrebreather Mask. A device used for a patient needing supplemental oxygen. It covers the nose and mouth.

NYPD. New York City Police Department.

PARAMEDIC, MEDIC, OR EMT-P. All titles have the same meaning. An advanced medical professional who delivers basic and advanced life support in the prehospital setting.

PAPD. Port Authority of New York and New Jersey Police Department.

PD. Pronounced pee-dee. Police Department.

THE PILE. A name given for Ground Zero after the rescue effort was discontinued.

PROTOCOLS. Standardized treatments for specific illness or injury within the paramedic's scope of practice.

RMP. Radio Motor Patrol. A squad car. It is what the earliest police cars equipped with two-way radios were called.

SCOTT PACK. An air tank carried by firefighters to allow them to breath in a smoke filled environment.

SECRET SQUIRREL. Street slang for a person who acts a little crazy. A name given for a paranoid EDP. Their usual dwelling place is the subway system of Manhattan. They emerge from the depths below when they feel that it is safe.

STANDING ORDERS. A set of medical treatments and drugs that paramedics may dispense without calling telemetry. A paramedic can give dozens of drugs on standing orders. For example: giving the drug Narcan for a patient in opiate overdose.

TECH. An ambulance crew consists of a "tech" (technician) who is mainly responsible for patient care and paperwork, and an MVO (motor vehicle operator), who is responsible for driving and taking care of the ambulance. The MVO is usually the senior medic.

TELEMETRY. Online medical control staffed by doctors who can give authorization for discretionary orders and protocol medical control options.

10-4. EMS radio code for "message is acknowledged."

10-6. EMS radio code for "stand-by."

10-13. NYPD radio code, used also by EMS. It means that an officer, paramedic or EMT needs emergency assistance.

10-55. Or fifty-five. NYPD radio code for "EMS call and no police are needed." The EMS personnel can release a police officer from the scene. Usually given to members of the NYPD or FDNY by EMS personnel when the former are not needed on a call.

10-63. Or sixty-three. EMS radio code for "a unit is responding to a given location or incident."

10-81. Or eighty-one. EMS radio code for "an ambulance unit has arrived at the hospital."

10-82. Or eighty-two. EMS radio code for "an ambulance unit enroute to the hospital."

10-83. Or eighty-three. EMS radio code for "a patient is pronounced dead on the scene."

10-85. Or eighty-five. NYPD radio code for "an additional unit is needed at the location and there is no emergency." Also used by EMS.

10-88. Or eighty-eight. EMS radio code for "an ambulance unit has arrived on the scene."

10-89. Or eighty-nine. EMS radio code for "an ambulance unit is at its assigned location."

10-90. Or ninety. EMS radio code for "an incident is unfounded or false alarm."

10-97. Or ninety-seven. EMS radio code for "an ambulance unit is available within its battalion."

10-98. Or ninety-eight. EMS radio code for "an ambulance unit is available but is outside of its battalion."

THE TOWERS. The Twin Towers. The World Trade Center.

TRIAGE. Means "sorting" in French. It is a way to separate patients and classify them according to the extent of their injuries. The most seriously injured are given immediate medical care or transport.

VOLUNTARY HOSPITALS. Noncity hospitals that operate in the 911 system of the City of New York. They provide hospital-based paramedics and EMTs. The majority of paramedics in the 911 system are hospital-based.

acknowledgements

This book has been a journey of the heart. At first it served
as my critical stress debriefing. It developed into first-hand
account of the brave people whose experiences I have shared on
a daily basis. This book is my way of thanking them for letting
me be part of their lives, sharing their victories, and being with
them in their time of sorrow.

In a project such as this, there are a great many people involved
whom I would like to thank:

First, I thank the president of the Princeton Book Company,
Charles H. Woodford, and his staff including my editor, Connie
Woodford. Charles' continued belief in this work, creative
suggestions, editing, and nurturing have made this book possible.
He is not only great at what he does; he is an exceptionally
sensitive human being.

Second, I would like to thank my friend and adviser Sean
Cassidy. The generosity with which he gave his time and talent
gave me the encouragement to continue the work and see it to
its completion.

I would especially like to thank Tara Cornetto and Todd
Ellison. They are my friends for life. Thanks to my agent, Leo
Bookman, of the Acme Talent and Literary Agency.

Thanks to all of my dear friends and co-workers, the
paramedics and supervisors of St. Vincent's Hospital in

acknowledgements

Manhattan, the nurses, doctors, residents, interns, technicians and clerks that make up our ER staff, and especially to Medical Director Dr. Richard Westfal, whose support and encouragement during the past three years is immeasurable.

Thanks to the NYPD, the PAPD and the greatest fire department in history, the FDNY—with special thanks to FDNY EMS Chief Robert A. McCracken. His leadership and bravery guided all of us through 9/11 and beyond. He is in every sense a caring and fair leader of all the men and women under his command.

Thanks to the Regional Emergency Medical Services Council, whose responsibility has been to coordinate the emergency medical services of the City of New York.

I would like also to thank Joseph Davis, EMT-P, the Emergency Services Coordinator of St. Vincent Catholic Medical Centers and Director of the Ambulance Department of St. Vincent's, Manhattan. He is the driving force behind St. Vincent's paramedics.

My heartfelt thanks and respect to the police officers, firefighters, EMS lieutenants and EMTs of Lower Manhattan who assist us on our medical calls.

I have the utmost gratitude and respect for my partner Steven Trautman. He is the smartest paramedic I know and the best friend I ever had. Also for my regular partners Scott Phelps and George Lindgren, two of the most caring and intelligent men I have ever known. And for my "Band of Brothers" on the night shift: Raquel Nery, Eric "Powder" Jiminez, Brian Saddler, Phil Eguiguiurens, Tony Montesino, and Charles Chinnici. During downtime they always understood while I worked on

acknowledgements

my rewrites and were a constant source of encouragement throughout this project.

I would like to acknowledge all of my teachers, those individuals who made a difference in my life. Most of all, I wish to acknowledge John DeLuca, my acting teacher, and Leon Portnoy, my first music teacher. Both are gentlemen of the highest caliber and the kindest nature.

Thanks to the United States Marine Corps and to my drill instructors at Parris Island, who gave me the tools to live my life and never quit.

To my Church and the priests who helped shape the way I think, and when I am at my best, the way I behave. My teachers and father confessors, Monsignor Lawrence McAlister, Father John (John Cardinal O'Connor), Father Paul Lazor, Father Thomas Hopko, Father Benedict Groeschel, CFR, Father John Breck, and Father John Meyendorff.

Finally, I would like to thank my family. My mother, Concetta Rella, drew the initial maps for the book and offered her comments. She also taught me to always hold my ground and try to do the right thing. Her example gave me the courage to face the impossible without fear. Special thanks goes to my brother Richard Rella, who clarified the direction of the book for me and so many times put me on the right path in life. To Tammy Rella, who proofread every version of the manuscript and never judged what I wrote. She is still the most courageous person I have ever known, and in every sense, has always been my better half.

about the author

Francis Rella was a member of the United States Marine Corps during the late 1970s and volunteered for service in the United States Navy Reserve during Operation Desert Shield. He served in the Navy as a Hospital Corpsman during the Gulf War and again volunteered for active service on September 13, 2001 after the attack on America.

He was on duty September 11 in Lower Manhattan and served at the World Trade Center throughout that day. He witnessed first-hand the collapse of both towers and he was the closest ambulance unit stationed under Building Seven when it collapsed.

He is a Nationally Registered Emergency Medical Technician–Paramedic serving in the EMS 911 system of the City of New York. He also holds New York City and New York State certification as a paramedic.

Rella has OSHA certification in Hazardous Materials Operations Training and is a Hazmat Team Leader at St. Vincent Catholic Medical Centers in New York City. He was promoted to paramedic supervisor in 2002.

Rella spent six years studying for the priesthood, which is the subject of a book now in progress. He holds a bachelor's degree and a master's degree in music. He has taught in both high school and college. While continuing to work as a paramedic he is pursuing a degree in nursing.

As a stage actor he has worked with such companies as the New York City Opera, the Light Opera of Manhattan and a number of summer stock and regional theaters. He is a member of Actor's Equity, Screen Actor's Guild, AGMA and AFTRA. In addition to his twenty years of professional experience as an actor, Rella is an award–winning radio writer. He produced and wrote the PBS radio mini-series "Great American Musicals," which was number one in its market. It later became a regular weekly program called "Opening Nights," running for another twelve years. He has written television scripts and has completed his first screenplay.

DATE

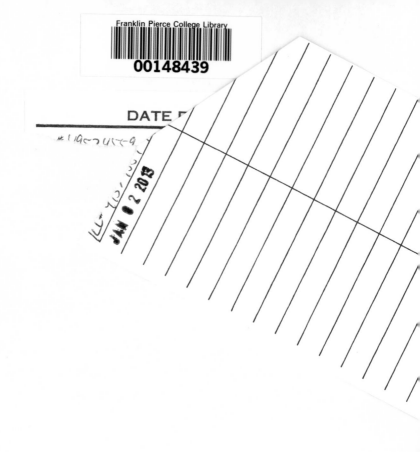